Praise for
Keeping Love Alive as Memories Fade

Through stories that are moving and unflinching, *Keeping Love Alive as Memories Fade* shows how love can persist even as dementia gradually erodes memory and physical abilities. It offers powerful testimony to the lasting nature and immense power of human relationships.

PETER V. RABINS, MD, MPH | Coauthor, *The 36-Hour Day*

Ed's personal and professional stories will resonate with caring couples and families desperately seeking reminders of the transformative resilience of loving long-term relationships. Long overdue, this book reminds families that although they don't have to do it all, meaningful connections can make a difference in the quality of family life despite progressive cognitive decline.

LISA P. GWYTHER, MSW, LCSW | Director, Duke (Alzheimer's) Family Support Program, Duke Health, and coauthor, *The Alzheimer's Action Plan*

Love lives on during times of loss, and there is profound value and redemption in intentionally expressing both the love and the grief that is part of the Alzheimer's journey. Yes! Be open. Be kind. The world needs more compassionate, love-affirming books like this.

ALAN D. WOLFELT, PHD | Director of the Center for Loss and Life Transition and author of *Healing Your Grieving Heart When Someone You Care About Has Alzheimer's*

As a geriatrician, I am all too familiar with Alzheimer's disease and the devastating effect it can have upon those afflicted and those who care for them. Alzheimer's and other dementias are the most terrifying complications of growing older, more feared than cancer, heart disease, and even death itself. So whether you simply wish to know more about these increasingly epidemic disorders, or especially if you are already dealing with their losses and challenges in yourself or a loved one, *Keeping Love Alive as Memories Fade* should be required reading. Artfully crafted and compellingly written, this compact volume brings hope, insight, and practical coping strategies into clear focus. For indeed love is the answer, and its flame must be kept alight through every phase of this journey to its end.

WILLIAM R. HAZZARD, MD | Professor of Internal Medicine, Section on Gerontology and Geriatric Medicine, Wake Forest School of Medicine, Wake Forest Baptist Health

Brilliant minds come together in this essential guide through the Alzheimer's journey! I would have loved this book when my mom was fading away. Real-life examples help you learn how to stay connected with the loved one you are watching disappear; specific daily exercises and tactics can help you stay in touch and in love. This roadmap of the Alzheimer's brain allows you to follow along, adapting and changing your interaction with a brain that is continuously changing with each stage of this disease. You can't fix what is breaking, but you can break through . . . with unconditional love.

LANIE POPE | Chief Meteorologist, WXII News, Winston-Salem, NC

A much-needed and refreshingly instructive guide devoted to the essential discussion of relationship, intimacy, and the complexities of connection at all stages in the dementia experience. Many wise books counsel caregivers on learning the language of dementia, but in the illuminating text of *Keeping Love Alive as Memories Fade*, the authors remind us of our deeply rooted shared humanity with persons with dementia, and that learning the transformative language of love is indeed the most profound, affirming, and enduring form of communication.

LISA SNYDER, MSW, LCSW | University of California, San Diego Author, *Speaking Our Minds: What It's Like to Have Alzheimer's*

KEEPING LOVE ALIVE AS MEMORIES FADE

The 5 Love Languages® and the Alzheimer's Journey

Deborah Barr, MA, MCHES, RHEd
Edward G. Shaw, MD, MA
GARY CHAPMAN, PhD

NORTHFIELD PUBLISHING | CHICAGO

Scripture quotations taken from the Amplified® Bible (AMPC), copyright © 1954, 1958, 1962, 1964, 1965, 1987 by The Lockman Foundation. Used by permission. www.Lockman.org.

Edited by Elizabeth Cody Newenhuyse
Interior design: Erik M. Peterson
Gary Chapman photo: P.S. Photography
Debbie Barr and Edward Shaw photos: Alysia Grimes
Cover design: Connie Gabbert Design and Illustration

Library of Congress Cataloging-in-Publication Data
Names: Chapman, Gary D.- author. | Barr, Deborah, author. | Shaw, Edward G., author.
Title: Keeping love alive as memories fade : the 5 love languages® and the Alzheimer's journey / Gary Chapman, PhD, Deborah Barr, MA, MCHES, Edward G. Shaw, MD, MA.
Description: Chicago : Northfield Publishing, [2016] | Includes bibliographical references.
Identifiers: LCCN 2016028240 (print) | LCCN 2016035160 (ebook) | ISBN 9780802414502 | ISBN 9780802494412 ()
Subjects: LCSH: Alzheimer's disease--Patients--Care.
Classification: LCC RC523 .C45 2016 (print) | LCC RC523 (ebook) | DDC 616.8/31--dc23
LC record available at https://lccn.loc.gov/2016028240

ISBN: 978-0-8024-1450-2

We hope you enjoy this book from Northfield Publishing. Our goal is to provide high-quality, thought-provoking books and products that connect truth to your real needs and challenges. For more information on other books and products that will help you with all your important relationships, go to 5lovelanguages.com or write to:

Northfield Publishing
820 N. LaSalle Boulevard
Chicago, IL 60610

1 3 5 7 9 10 8 6 4 2

Printed in the United States of America

Dedicated to Rebecca Easterly Shaw,
loving daughter, sister, wife, mother, and friend

Contents

About the Authors

Gary Chapman, PhD, has been a pastor and marriage counselor for more than 35 years. He is the author of the book that inspired this one: *The 5 Love Languages®: The Secret to Love That Lasts,* which has now sold over 10 million copies worldwide and has been translated into 50 languages. A prolific writer, Gary has also authored *Love Languages* editions for men, singles, and parents, as well as numerous books on marriage, anger, apology, and other topics. He speaks to thousands of couples across the country through weekend marriage conferences and hosts two nationally syndicated radio programs. As the originator of the five love languages, Gary's insights on the expression of love in human relationships undergird each chapter.

Deborah Barr, MA, MCHES, is a master certified health education specialist and journalist. An experienced wellness writer, Debbie brought a health educator's perspective to numerous aspects of the book, including the detrimental health effects of long-term caregiving and the looming Alzheimer's disease epidemic. Her familiarity with the love languages is longstanding, having provided editorial support for Gary as he wrote the original *5 Love Languages* book. While working as clinic coordinator for the Memory Counseling Program at Wake Forest Baptist

Medical Center, she learned that Ed Shaw was incorporating the five love languages into his dementia counseling—and the idea for this book was born. As the lead writer and information gatherer for the team, the book is primarily written in her "voice." Like Drs. Chapman and Shaw, she resides in Winston-Salem, North Carolina. This is her fourth book.

Edward G. Shaw, MD, MA, is dually trained as a physician and a mental health counselor. He is the primary care partner for his wife, Rebecca, who was diagnosed with early-onset Alzheimer's disease at age 53. He was a practicing radiation oncologist for 23 years and a world-renowned brain tumor expert. In 2010, inspired by Rebecca's journey, his medical interest shifted to dementia diagnosis and treatment, and with his additional training in mental health and grief counseling, he founded the Memory Counseling Program that is now part of Wake Forest Baptist Health in Winston-Salem, North Carolina. A career cognitive function researcher, Ed's expertise on brain anatomy, function, and mental health diagnosis and treatment were invaluable assets to this project. His moving personal story of caring for his wife, coupled with his innovative use of the five love languages in dementia counseling, inspired the central message of the book.

Foreword

I CANNOT ADEQUATELY express my heartfelt endorsement of this book, and I know that you will find it equally moving. Writing this foreword was difficult for me because, as is chronicled in chapter 1, Ed and Rebecca Shaw (Becky, as I know her) and their daughters, Erin, Leah, and Carrie, were once my next-door neighbors. Our families grew up together. I and my family—my wife, Diane, and our children, Lindsay and Matt—were best friends with the Shaw family.

After the Shaws had relocated to North Carolina, when Ed called me to express his concern about Rebecca's memory at age 53, I could not believe it. Ed and Rebecca traveled to Rochester so I could evaluate Rebecca. Sadly, the evaluation confirmed that this relatively young, bright, and devoted person was in fact beginning her journey with Alzheimer's disease.

With that as background, I would like to say that Ed and his coauthors, Deborah Barr and Dr. Gary Chapman, have penned what I believe to be the most emotionally laden, yet extremely insightful book about the relationship challenges that families must navigate during the painful course of Alzheimer's disease.

I have never encountered a more dedicated soulmate and caregiver than Ed, who left a successful career as an academic radiation oncologist to devote his life to caring for his Rebecca. Along the way, he acquired additional professional training in mental health and dementia care in order to help others who are traveling the same path. The result is this work, built upon Ed's love for Rebecca and counseling experience, Deborah's expertise as a health educator, and Gary's framework of the five love languages, yielding practical advice for spouses, family caregivers, and health care providers involved in the care of those with Alzheimer's and other dementias.

With love as its primary theme, *Keeping Love Alive as Memories Fade: The 5 Love Languages® and the Alzheimer's Journey* is an invaluable resource for caregivers from all walks of life. It describes strategies for maintaining an emotional bond with a person who has dementia while preserving the individual's dignity and self-respect throughout the disease. This book also well describes the sacrificial nature of caregiving, offers a simple framework for addressing challenging behaviors, and provides basic information about the brain and how it changes over the course of the disease.

If she were able to read this book, Rebecca would be proud of what she inspired. This wonderful work is entirely consistent with the kind of person she is.

RONALD C. PETERSEN, MD, PhD
Professor of Neurology
Cora Kanow Professor of Alzheimer's Disease Research
Distinguished Mayo Clinic Investigator
Director, Mayo Clinic Alzheimer's Disease Research Center
Director, Mayo Clinic Study of Aging
Mayo Clinic College of Medicine
Rochester, MN

A Word from Gary

WHEN DEBBIE CONTACTED me about working with her and Dr. Shaw in writing this book, I was immediately interested. Interested first because I was thrilled to hear that Dr. Shaw had been using *The 5 Love Languages*® in his counseling with those who were walking the Alzheimer's journey. Secondly, I was interested because, as a pastoral counselor, I have counseled many families who have taken this unwanted journey. On the personal side, I have watched my brother-in-law, who was a brilliant university professor, steadily decline to late-stage Alzheimer's disease. I have felt deeply for his wife who kept him at home as long as she could and then made the hard decision to place him in a long-term care facility. Their adult children have experienced the grief of the pre-death loss of their dad.

I have been very encouraged as I have sat in on several of Dr. Shaw's support groups for caregivers. Most of these groups have been composed of spouses of the Alzheimer's patients. Their dedication to intentional, sacrificial love has amazed me. The smiles on their faces when they receive a small, loving response from their spouses reflect their deep satisfaction in what they are doing. Then, when the patient is no longer capable of responding, to see their spouses choosing to continue expressing love in all five languages hoping that, at least for a moment, they will feel loved, is so rewarding. One wife said, "I continue loving for myself as much as for my husband. When the end comes, I want to look back and have no regrets."

Almost everyone agrees that the deepest emotional need we have is the need to love and be loved. When one becomes incapable of giving love, I believe they are still capable of receiving love. I first discovered this in the nursing home where my mother lived the last year of her life. When I would walk down the hallway lined with wheelchairs, those who occupied those chairs would reach out with their arms and make unintelligible sounds. When I responded by bending over and hugging them, they would "melt in my arms." I would speak affirming words to them and their spirit would calm down, and at least for that moment, life was beautiful. Later, I encountered a chaplain who sang to patients who were no longer verbal. Amazingly, some of them would start tapping their feet to the beat of the music, and some even sang the words with him. They could not speak, but the music touched something in the brain that responded.

It is interesting that so many of those caregivers, who demonstrated intentional, sacrificial love for their family member who was suffering from the results of Alzheimer's disease, had a strong faith in God. More than one said, "I could not make it without God and my church family." I am convinced that God wants everyone to experience His love and then to share that love with all whom we encounter. By nature, we are selfish—we love those who love us. When we receive God's love, we are empowered to love even those who do not, or cannot, love us. This is the love that I have seen demonstrated by so many caregivers.

When I discovered the concept of the five love languages in

my counseling practice, I never dreamed that the original book would sell over 10 million copies in English, and be translated into over 50 languages around the world. The series of books that followed, *The 5 Love Languages® of Children* and versions for teenagers, singles, men, and military couples, have helped millions of people express love more effectively in their marriage, parenting, and friendships. I never thought about its application to the Alzheimer's journey. However, I am excited to see how this book will help those who walk this un-chosen road. If you find the book helpful, I hope you will share it with your friends who walk a similar path.

Gary Chapman, PhD
Winston-Salem, NC

1

Ed and Rebecca: A Love Story

IT WAS A BEAUTIFUL North Carolina morning in August 2013. Rebecca and I (Ed) were sipping our coffee on the back porch, part of our morning ritual. Without warning, the awful moment I had long dreaded finally arrived. Rebecca looked at me and said, "I have no idea who you are." Her blank stare confirmed that she really meant it.

"But Sweetie, I am your husband, Ed. You are my wife. We've been married for 33 years." This clue, more like a plea, didn't help. The pain of the moment drove me from the porch into the house. Tears streaming down my face, I stood before our family portrait, taken only months before, at Thanksgiving. I looked into the faces of our daughter, Erin, her husband, Darian, their two-year-old son, Paul, our other daughters, Leah and Carrie, sweet Rebecca, and me. I was overcome with the need to talk to one of the girls. I reached Leah first. When she answered, there were no words, just sobs, deep sobs that started in my feet and shook my body as they reached for my heart, landing in my eyes, which streamed like a leaky faucet.

"Mama has forgotten us. We're gone."

Many times I've reflected back on that terrible morning, asking myself the same unanswerable question: how could 37 years of a loving relationship and a third of a century of marriage disappear from Rebecca's mind overnight?

Rebecca Lynn Easterly and I began dating in the fall of 1976. We were students at the University of Iowa, where we both were sophomores, she a speech pathology major, I, premed. I asked her out on my 19th birthday, October 30th. She was sitting in the student union studying over a cup of coffee, and she was beautiful. Silky-smooth blonde hair, long legs, a blue leotard top, bellbottom jeans, and a face that radiated kindness. We had met briefly the year before. I hoped she'd remember me. After getting up the nerve to reintroduce myself, she accepted my invitation for our first date. One week later we went dancing and had dinner at the Brown Bottle, an iconic Iowa City restaurant. During dinner and afterwards, we talked and talked and talked. We had so much in common. Although we both had alcoholic fathers, we shared a love of family, especially children, and an appreciation for nature as a reflection of the Creator's hand (though at the time, I was a committed agnostic). I walked her home, we shared our first kiss, and we both knew that we were in love. Three weeks later, we talked about marriage and the desire to have three children, all daughters. Three and a half years later, we were married.

> How could 37 years of a loving relationship disappear from Rebecca's mind overnight?

Rebecca graduated summa cum laude with a near-4.0 GPA, in the top 1 percent of her graduating class. She later received a master's degree in speech pathology from Iowa. After completing my premed studies, I went to medical school at Rush Medical College in Chicago. In May 1983, we headed north to the Mayo Clinic in Rochester, Minnesota, three-week-old Erin in tow. There, I completed my internship and residency in radiation oncology and remained as an attending physician, launching a career as a brain tumor doctor. Our second daughter, Leah, was born in 1985, and three years later Carrie completed the trio of daughters we had dreamed of during our courtship. We spent 12 years in Rochester, happy and surrounded by family and friends.

In 1995, we headed southeast to Winston-Salem, North Carolina and the Wake Forest School of Medicine for an offer too good to refuse: a radiation oncology chairmanship and the opportunity to establish a research program in how brain cancer and its treatments affect brain **cognitive function** (words in bold type are defined at the end of the chapter). We thrived as Southerners. Erin, Leah, and Carrie marched through the ranks of elementary, middle, and high school, and then college. Throughout those years, Rebecca was "supermom." Navigating with her Day Planner notebook, kindness, and grace, she organized, fed, and nurtured our family while I was busy seeing patients, publishing journal articles, teaching, and getting research grants.

In the spring of 2005, as our family was preparing with excitement for Erin and Darian's wedding, Erin noticed something odd: her "super mom" was struggling to keep up with the details of wedding planning. It all came together, though, and in May we celebrated the marriage of our oldest daughter. One year later, we mourned when Rebecca's older sister, Leslie, died from colon cancer. This was the first tragedy our extended family had experienced. Rebecca was deeply saddened by Leslie's death, as she and Leslie had been kindred spirits. Throughout the summer, fall, and winter of 2006 and the spring of 2007, Rebecca was sad. She was distant, a bit disorganized, and forgetful. I attributed it to grief and a gradually emptying nest, until one Saturday morning as we sat, me reading the newspaper, Rebecca the latest issue of *U.S. News and World Report*. Rebecca said, "I've read this article three times and I can't remember a thing about what it says." At her age, 53, I knew this was not normal.

One day the following week, my car was in the shop. Rebecca was going to pick me up from work at 5:30 p.m. and take me to the dealership to retrieve my car. Usually prompt, she hadn't arrived on time. At 6:00, I called her, a bit miffed. "Are you going to pick me up?" She had no idea she was supposed to come and get me.

"Okay, I'm on my way," she said.

We lived only 10 minutes from the medical center, but she didn't arrive until 6:30.

"What took so long?" I inquired.

"Oh, I took a different way of getting here."

When she described her route, I realized that she'd gotten lost along the way. I had always marveled at Rebecca's sense of direction, and had even nicknamed her "the human compass." Now I was really worried.

Wake Forest School of Medicine is well known for both geriatric research and care. In mid-2007, I made an appointment for Rebecca to see Dr. Jeff Williamson, head of geriatrics and a well-known **dementia** expert. In his initial assessment, Dr. Williamson diagnosed Rebecca with depression and prescribed an antidepressant.

"Let's see if things improve after a couple of months on the medication. Depression is a common cause of memory loss." But

I could tell he was worried that something more was going on. So was I.

After her symptoms failed to improve, Dr. Williamson decided to order some blood tests, a magnetic resonance imaging (MRI) scan of Rebecca's brain, and assess some of her **cognitive functions** such as attention, memory, language, multitasking, and spatial skills. The blood tests came back normal, but the MRI showed mild shrinkage of Rebecca's brain, especially in the regions that control memory and spatial skills. The cognitive assessment confirmed loss of short-term memory and spatial skills way out of proportion with what would be expected for Rebecca's age and educational level.

Dr. Williamson told us, "My diagnosis is something called **mild cognitive impairment (MCI)**, a condition that often leads to Alzheimer's disease. I think you should get a second opinion. Rebecca is too young to have Alzheimer's, especially since she doesn't have any family history of the disease."

Our next-door neighbor in Rochester, Minnesota had been a Mayo Clinic neurologist named Ronald Petersen. He and his wife, Diane, had two children who were about the same ages as our girls. Diane and Rebecca often carpooled, as our kids went to the same elementary school. Affectionately known to us as "RP," Dr. Petersen was a nationally and internationally recognized expert on Alzheimer's disease. In fact, it was his research that led to the discovery of MCI as a precursor to Alzheimer's. Getting a second opinion from him seemed logical. Not only was he "the best" dementia doctor in the world, he had known Rebecca for 20 years.

In the early summer of 2008, we spent a week at the Mayo Clinic where Rebecca had an extensive evaluation to find the cause of her memory loss. In addition to blood tests, a spinal tap, and more in-depth neuropsychological testing, Dr. Peterson ordered a special MRI scan and two Positron Emission Tomography (PET) scans. One PET scan was done to reveal Rebecca's brain metabolism; the other, a newer type of PET scan, was done to reveal amyloid, a protein that collects abnormally in the brain, causing inflammation, deterioration, and shrinkage. Amyloid and another protein, tau, form the **"plaques and tangles"** that are thought to cause the brain damage of Alzheimer's disease.

Despite our earnest hopes and fervent prayers to the contrary, the diagnosis was definitive: **early-onset Alzheimer's disease**. The prognosis: 8–10 years' life expectancy, progressive decline in all brain functions, the need for professional caregivers, and possibly nursing home placement.

> We embraced as we cried, speaking our love for one another in silence.

After receiving the news, Rebecca and I drove in silence to the Minneapolis airport to catch our return flight home. We wept as we drove, exchanging glances filled with sadness, fear, and uncertainty. At Pine Island, a small town north of Rochester where Rebecca had worked as an elementary school speech teacher, I pulled over. We had to talk. Rebecca asked me, "What does this mean for us? For the girls?" She had already forgotten what Dr. Petersen said, so I told her again. We then embraced as we cried, speaking our love for one another in silence, reaffirming the vows we had made to each other 28 years earlier.

Her voice full of sadness, Rebecca said, "I don't want to be a

ED AND REBECCA: A LOVE STORY

burden. I want Erin, Leah, and Carrie to live their lives, pursue their dreams and not let this get in the way. I will be okay. I know God loves me and will take care of me. Eternity in heaven is as real to me as life on this earth." This was the only time we would ever directly speak about her Alzheimer's.

In the years that followed, Rebecca's dementia progressed relentlessly through the stages of Alzheimer's disease. By the spring of 2010, her driving skills had deteriorated to the point that she was no longer safe on the road in her bright red Volkswagen Beetle. Navigating from home even to nearby destinations had become too challenging. On one occasion, a wrong turn took her several towns south of Winston-Salem, about 25 miles from home. Scratches mysteriously appeared on the side of the car. She drove very slowly, stopping in the middle of the road when she was unsure of where to go. Finally, the keys had to be taken away.

"I don't understand why I can't drive," she protested. "I've never gotten a ticket nor have I been in an accident. It's unfair." Like so many people who have dementia, she didn't have insight into how the disease was slowly stealing her abilities, moving her toward disability.

Shortly after Rebecca had to give up her car keys, she and I took a driving trip to the Pocono Mountains. We made a stop at the Crayola factory, which brought back warm memories of Rebecca and our daughters coloring around the kitchen table when they were younger. What we had hoped would be a fun adventure turned sour when Rebecca left her purse under a bench while we watched a demonstration on how crayons are made. Unfortunately, we didn't realize that the purse was missing until after the Crayola factory had closed. We spent the night nearby and went back in the morning, but the purse was nowhere to be found. We filed a police report and left. This incident upset Rebecca immensely.

"I hate my brain," she said, teary-eyed, as we drove away.

Later that summer, while walking to the grocery store, Rebecca got lost. As she was about to turn onto one of the busiest north-south streets in the city, Elizabeth, a family friend, just happened to be driving by and saw Rebecca looking at street signs. It was obvious that Rebecca was trying to figure out where she was. Elizabeth pulled over, lowered her window, and called to Rebecca, "Where are you headed?"

"To the grocery store," Rebecca replied.

"Jump in. I'll give you a ride," Elizabeth offered, realizing that Rebecca was walking in the opposite direction of the store.

To this day, our family thinks of Elizabeth as a guardian angel, and we wonder what might have happened if she hadn't been in that place at that time.

Shortly after the grocery store incident, we hired Rebecca's first paid caregiver. Erica, a certified nursing assistant (CNA), spent the weekdays companioning Rebecca on her journey with Alzheimer's disease. Within four years, Rebecca would require round-the-clock caregivers. This crew—affectionately known as the "A-team" (because their names, Letisa, Fatima, Tasha, and Florina all end in "a," as does Rebecca)—is still with us, caring for Rebecca day and night.

Looking back, I would have to say that the most difficult and challenging days of Rebecca's Alzheimer's journey were the four months that followed the awful day in 2013 when she "lost" the girls and me. She became very agitated, especially starting at dusk and on into the early evening (known as **"sundowning"**).

"I want to go home," she'd say, marching around the house

from door to door, trying to escape.

"But you are home, Sweetie," I would tell her. "This is our home."

She could not be comforted. Rebecca was yearning for her childhood home, a small bungalow in her hometown of Cedar Rapids, Iowa, where she had lived in the mid-to-late 1960s. I would have to physically block her attempts to exit as she punched and kicked at me, behaviors that were so atypical for sweet and gentle Rebecca. Dr. Williamson prescribed a medication that reduced some of Rebecca's aggression, but caused her to become withdrawn and deeply depressed. During this time she would lie on her bed or the couch and sob inconsolably. Dr. Williamson then tried a different medication which, over time, reduced her agitation and returned her mood to normal and helped her sleep.

After Rebecca no longer recognized me as her husband, we continued to sleep in the same bed, but she turned her back to me and stayed on the very edge of the bed, as far away as she could be without falling out. One night she became very agitated and told me she didn't want me sleeping in the same bed as her, so I set up a twin daybed in the corner of our bedroom. Those first few nights I was sleepless, grieving. We were only separated by a few feet, but it felt as though she were a million miles away.

Early in our marriage, Rebecca and I discovered we both fell asleep more easily if we were touching one another, either by "spooning," facing in the same direction with my one arm wrapped around her, or turning opposite of one another, "rump to rump." Sometimes we wouldn't go right off to sleep. Rather, we'd make love, then spend some time together in one another's arms, talking about how blessed we were to have each other and to have Erin, Leah, and Carrie. For the first couple of months of being alone at night in the twin bed, I would lie awake, literally aching with the desire to touch Rebecca, to lie in bed with her, to hold her. During these months I had several long conversations with God, thanking Him for bringing Rebecca and me together as husband and wife, for blessing us with amazing children, but in the same breath asking how I could love this woman without being able to touch her. With this loss I began my own journey of loneliness and celibacy.

> We were only separated by a few feet, but it felt as though she were a million miles away.

In early 2014, I moved into my own bedroom since Rebecca was getting up multiple times during the night and I found it impossible to get enough sleep to function at work. She had no concept of the day, date, month, season, or year. She was unable to read or write, even to sign her own name, or add two plus two. Another challenge was spatial orientation. She had lost the ability to center her bottom over a chair or couch and required assistance just to sit, including sitting on the toilet. With these further declines, evening and nighttime caregivers were added to the A-team. This meant that Rebecca and I would never again have an evening alone at home together. There didn't seem to be any part of our lives that Alzheimer's disease hadn't taken away or changed.

In the two years since then, Rebecca has transitioned into late-stage Alzheimer's disease. She lives only in the moment with no remembrance of the past and no thought of the future. Her days are spent coloring at the kitchen table, putting simple puzzles together, and breaking twigs into small pieces. She initiates no conversation, speaks unintelligibly, and often needs to hear something repeated multiple times before she can understand what has been said to her. She walks slowly and unsteadily, always at risk for a fall. Because she is so unsteady, and also has difficulty processing visual information, someone must accompany and hold onto her at all times. Due to unpredictable urinary incontinence, she wears pull-up adult diapers. She needs help using the toilet, taking a shower, and getting dressed. Her medicines must be crushed and mixed into food as she cannot swallow pills any longer. Despite all this, she is happy most of the time.

Though she doesn't acknowledge me as her husband, at some level I am familiar to her. At the very least, I'm the nice man who lives in the same house that she does. My love for her is unaltered. When I return home from work, my time is Rebecca's time. It is important to me that I make her supper and help her eat. The smile on her face when she is given her dessert—always ice cream in a cone or a dish—brings as much joy to me as it does to her. Afterward, we sit on the couch and watch old musicals on a DVD player. Her favorite is *The Sound of Music*, which we've watched together hundreds of times. For Rebecca, the familiarity of each song is comforting. For me, it is a time when we're physically close, perhaps holding hands, being present to one another. Bedtime is also a special time. After her caregivers prepare her for sleep and get her tucked in, I will spend five or ten minutes saying goodnight, our only alone time each day. She will let me kiss her on the cheek or forehead. I tell her, "I love you. I love you more than anyone else in the whole world. You are the best sweetie a man could have. And we're married. We've been married for 35 years. We have three daughters, Erin, Leah, and Carrie. They love you and know they have the best mommy ever. See you in the morning. Sleep tight and don't let the bedbugs bite" (something we always said to the girls). Sometimes, Rebecca will say thank you. Once in a while, she'll utter something that sounds like "I love you too." Most often, her eyes are closed and she is drifting off to sleep.

The Christmas 2015 season was a time when our entire family was together. We connected with Rebecca, loving her in as many ways as we could, and loved she was. Erin shared a good-morning hug and sat with Rebecca drinking her morning coffee, just as she had since high school. Leah played familiar songs on her guitar while she and Rebecca "sang" together. Carrie snuggled next to Rebecca on the couch, her head on Rebecca's shoulder. My favorite way to add to the fun was sneaking in some kisses on Rebecca's cheek and neck, which often made her giggle like a schoolgirl and say "yuck" as she wiped off the side of her face. Rebecca's mom visited with freshly baked cookies; her friends brought flowers; and her sister and sister-in-law came for a visit just to spend time with Rebecca. Her caregivers had their own ways of showing love: they brushed her hair, painted her nails, and brought her the gift of a beautiful new blouse. Even our grandson, Paul, was drawn to his grandmother, helping her put a simple puzzle together or sharing a marker and coloring on the same page with her. We chose, with intention, to experience the joy of Rebecca's presence, rather than dwelling on the possibility that this very well might be our last Christmas together as a complete family.

Rebecca is now in her ninth year on the Alzheimer's journey, and I don't know how much longer the journey will last. It has been a long, hard journey, emotionally, physically, and spiritually, and one that I wish we were not taking. Yet there are so many things I've learned, about Rebecca, about me, and about us, because of it. I know, if the situation had been reversed, me with dementia and Rebecca as my care partner, she would have taken care of me with the same level of commitment that I've had in caring for her. I also know that if I could somehow carry this burden for her, trade her diseased brain for my normal one, I'd do it without a second thought, just to know that she would be able to live to a ripe old age knowing those she's loved. If I had known before we married that she was going to develop early-onset Alzheimer's, I still would have married her in a heartbeat. The life we've had—now 40 years together, 36 of them married, three children, a son-in-law, and two grandsons—has been more than we could have ever dreamed. And I have learned, through the grace of God, to find an endless supply of love for Rebecca and to maintain emotional intimacy with her. I know that at some level, in her own way, she also loves me. And while the thought of losing her is unbearable to all who love her, we are comforted by the knowledge of her deep personal faith and the way she has lived her life because of it.

EDWARD G. SHAW
Winston-Salem, NC

Terms to Know

The bolded words that appear in Ed's story are defined and explained below, along with other terms and facts about Alzheimer's disease (AD). Understanding these key terms and facts will help you gain the most from the remaining chapters of this book.

Care Partner. The care partner is the primary person providing direct care to the person with dementia, most often a spouse or an adult child. In the United States, Canada, and China, most dementia-related resources and literature refer to this person as the *caregiver.* In some other countries, *carer* or *caretaker* is preferred. At the risk of bucking convention, throughout this book we have mainly used the term *care partner.* We prefer this term, especially in the early stages of AD, because it is less hierarchical, allowing the person with the disease to feel emotionally equal to the person providing care. Our observation is that family care partners tend to provide care with a sense of loyalty that aligns with the definition of *partner:* "a player on the same side or team as another" (dictionary.com). Thus, we are more comfortable applying the word *caregiver* to paid professionals than to family members. At the same time, we acknowledge that around the midpoint of the disease, care partnering transitions to a more truly care *giving* role.

Cognitive Function. The brain has five cognitive functions:

- Attention
- Memory and learning
- Language
- Executive (the ability to plan, solve problems, make decisions, and multitask)

▫ Visual-spatial (The *visual* aspect allows us to recognize faces; the *spatial* aspect is our internal "GPS"—the ability to perceive relationships between objects in our visual field.)

Alzheimer's disease is characterized by progressive difficulties in memory and learning, executive function, and visual-spatial function. By late-stage AD, however, all of the cognitive functions are affected.

Dementia. Dementia is not a specific disease, but rather an umbrella term for a wide range of symptoms related to memory loss, declining cognitive function, or changes in personality. There are many types of dementia. Alzheimer's disease is the most common type, accounting for 60–80 percent of all cases. Because most dementia is due to AD, it gets the most attention from both the media and the medical profession. Thanks to Lisa Genova's bestselling book, *Still Alice,* the award-winning movie by the same name, a plethora of TV pharmaceutical ads, and high-profile patients, such as President Ronald Reagan and singer Glen Campbell, almost everyone has now heard of Alzheimer's disease. For this reason, we have chosen to focus primarily on AD in this book. In the chapters ahead, the terms *Alzheimer's disease, AD,* and *dementia* are used interchangeably.

Early-onset Alzheimer's disease. The majority of individuals diagnosed with AD are 65 years of age or older (late-onset AD). Early-onset Alzheimer's disease, also called younger-onset Alzheimer's disease, starts before age 65, often affecting those in their 40s and 50s. Early-onset AD is uncommon, affecting only about 5 percent of those with AD (about 200,000 people in the United States).[1]

Mild cognitive impairment (MCI). MCI is the "gray area" between normal age-related memory loss and the memory loss of mild Alzheimer's disease. A person with MCI has more memory problems than others of their same age and educational level. They may find it hard to remember names, and may forget appointments or social events. They may have difficulty following the thread of a conversation, book, or movie. Decision-making or tasks that require planning may feel overwhelming. Subtle changes in the person's personality may be present. However, these problems are usually not serious enough to interfere with daily life. While MCI progresses to AD or another type of dementia about 70 percent of the time, some people never get worse, and a few will even eventually get better.

Plaques and Tangles. In 1906, Dr. Alois Alzheimer discovered two abnormal structures in the brains of people who had died of what we now know as Alzheimer's disease. Today, these abnormal structures are called "plaques and tangles." Plaques are deposits of beta-amyloid protein (or "amyloid"). Neurofibrillary tangles are twisted fibers of another protein, tau (rhymes with "now"). Amyloid plaques build up in the spaces *between* the brain's nerve cells (neurons); tau tangles build up *within* the neurons themselves. Most of us develop some plaques and tangles as we age; this is normal. People with AD, however, develop excessive amounts of these proteins, which hinder cell-to-cell communication and cause brain inflammation. Eventually, the toxic presence of plaques and tangles causes so much damage that nerve cells die. As plaques and tangles spread throughout the brain, widespread cell death occurs. As neurons die, the brain shrinks, resulting in memory and cognitive function loss, personality changes, and the progressive inability to carry out normal daily functions. The exact role of plaques and tangles is not clearly understood, but scientists do now know that amyloid may begin accumulating in the brain 10 to 20 years before the first symptom of forgetfulness appears.

PWD. Person with dementia. (You will see this abbreviation throughout the book.)

Sundowning. Sundowning is a state of confusion that typically begins at dusk and extends into the evening hours. Challenging behaviors may include agitation, aggression, anxiety, fear, pacing, and wandering. Some individuals express a yearning to "go home" to a time and place in the past, perhaps from childhood. The cause of sundowning is unknown. About 18 percent of those with AD experience sundowning.[2]

FACTS ABOUT ALZHEIMER'S DISEASE

- As of 2016, 5.4 million Americans have AD.
- One in nine Americans age 65 or older has AD. One-third of those age 85 and older have it.
- Older African Americans are twice as likely to get AD as older whites.
- Older Hispanics are about one and a half times as likely as older whites to get AD.
- Nearly two-thirds of those with AD are women.
- Age is the greatest risk factor for AD.
- Two-thirds of all dementia caregivers are women. Over half are adult children caring for parents.

- About 250,000 children between ages 8 and 18 help someone care for a person with AD or another dementia.
- At present, there is no way to prevent, cure, or slow the progression of Alzheimer's disease.

Source: Alzheimer's Association, *2016 Alzheimer's Disease Facts and Figures*[3]

2

Love: It's All in Your Head

"There is no substitute for the love of an
Alzheimer's caregiver."
—BOB DEMARCO

ALZHEIMER'S DISEASE does not just affect the diagnosed person, but the whole family; it is a family disease. While Ed and his daughters know this firsthand, from the sidelines we (Gary and Debbie) also compassionately acknowledge the relational separation and trauma created by this disease. AD severely challenges relationships, and is laden with potential to completely derail them. Indeed, not all friendships or family ties endure to the end of the Alzheimer's journey.

Ed sometimes describes the relational damage of AD as an unraveling tapestry. The beautiful design of a marriage, a family, or a friendship, so lovingly woven over the years, is slowly distorted as the disease relentlessly pulls at the fibers that once entwined to create it. Nothing can stop the unraveling; the disease is incurable. It is the mission of our book, however, to assert that the application of *intentional love* is powerful and beautiful, worth applying even to a tapestry that will inevitably fully unravel.

What does it mean to truly love someone? And what if, as is the case with AD, the person you love eventually becomes unable to express love back to you? We will explore these questions throughout the book. Our grounding perspective, however, is well captured in an excerpt from *The 5 Love Languages*®. In the third chapter, Gary wrote:

> Our most basic emotional need is not to fall in love but to be genuinely loved by another, to know a love that grows out of reason and choice, not instinct. I need to be loved by someone who chooses to love me, who sees in me something worth loving. That kind of love requires effort and discipline. It is the choice to expend energy in an effort to benefit the other person, knowing that if his or her life is enriched by your effort, you too will find a sense of satisfaction—the satisfaction of having genuinely loved another . . . [When] love is the attitude that says, ". . . I choose to look out for your interests" . . . the one who chooses to love will find appropriate ways to express that decision.

Love that is driven not by infatuation or obsession, but by choice, says Gary, is "real love."[1]

> What if the person you love eventually becomes unable to express love back to you?

The English word "love" does not adequately describe the depth and beauty of the choice-driven kind of love that Gary is talking about. The Hebrew language, however, has a word that does capture the full meaning of this truest form of love. The word is *hesed* (HEH-sed). Its meaning is a blend of love and loyalty. Because it has no English equivalent it has been translated in various ways, including kindness, steadfast love, loyalty, and faithfulness.[2] Author Lois Tverberg unpacked the riches of this word when she wrote that "*hesed* acts out of unswerving loyalty . . . *hesed* is love that can be counted on . . . It's not about the thrill of romance, but the security of faithfulness . . . Like other Hebrew words, *hesed* is not just a feeling but an action. It intervenes on behalf of loved ones and comes to their rescue."[3]

Our heartfelt wish is to encourage readers to choose and cultivate the intentional love described by *hesed*. It is this commitment to love by choice that empowers us, as Gary wrote, to "find appropriate ways to express that decision" in the relationally challenging context of AD.

THE FIVE LOVE LANGUAGES

The concept of intentional love has become operational for many people as they have gained an understanding of the five love languages. If you've read one of the *5 Love Languages*® books, maybe you have used its simple yet profound message to transform a relationship of your own. If so, perhaps you are now intrigued by the notion that the love languages can be used in the context of Alzheimer's disease to keep love alive even as a person's memories are fading. If you are not already familiar with the five love languages, we encourage you to read or listen to one of the books (see Appendix C for a list of these titles).

Whether you are familiar with the love languages or not, before we apply them in the context of Alzheimer's disease, here's a brief recap to give us all a common framework:

Imagine how difficult it would be to communicate with someone from China if you did not know a word of Chinese and he did not know a word of English. You could draw pictures or point at words in a dictionary or physically act out your message, but to really communicate effectively, at least one of you would have to learn to speak the other person's language. In *The 5 Love Languages*®, Gary used the metaphor of literal languages to help readers understand that the ways individuals perceive emotional love are so distinct from one another that they essentially comprise five different "languages" or channels of communication.[4] Each of us has at least one language that communicates emotional love to us more than the others.

Gary defines the five love languages as:

> ***Words of Affirmation*:** unsolicited compliments, whether verbal or written, or words of appreciation. Examples: "I love you." "You did an amazing job!" "You look great in that dress." "I really appreciate your attention to details." "Dialects" include words of encouragement, humble words, and words of kindness. Saying nice things about a person to others counts too because the message often travels back to him or her as others repeat the compliment. A *"Words of Affirmation* person" can be emotionally devastated by insults and harsh words.

> ***Quality Time*:** giving someone your full, undivided attention. Dialects are quality conversation (sharing thoughts, feelings, desires, and experiences, with the emphasis on really listening to another person) and quality activities (sharing memory-making experiences). A *"Quality Time*

person" can be hurt by halfhearted or distracted listening, or by repeatedly postponing promised time together.

Gifts (or "Receiving Gifts"): any purchased, handmade, or found tangible gift to let someone know you care. A gift is a visible symbol of love. Price is irrelevant—meaningful gifts can range from costly to having no monetary value at all. It is the thoughtfulness and effort behind a gift that sends the "I love you" message. Being physically present, the gift of your time, is an intangible gift that is very precious to some people, especially in times of crisis, illness, or celebration. A *"Gifts* person" can be hurt by a forgotten anniversary or birthday, or left feeling empty in a relationship void of tangible tokens of love.

Acts of Service: doing helpful things for another person, such as setting the table, walking the dog, washing dishes, vacuuming, or grocery shopping. The purpose of *Acts of Service* is to lighten the load of the other person. Acts of service require thought, planning, time, and effort. The idea is not simply to stay busy, or to do the tasks *you* enjoy most, but to do the things that are most meaningful and helpful to the *other* person. An *"Acts of Service* person" can be hurt by laziness, someone leaving a mess for them to clean up, or forgotten promises to help.

Physical Touch: deliberate touch that requires your full attention to deliver, such as a back rub, a foot massage, a hug, a "high five," or a kiss; incidental touch that requires little or no extra investment of time, such as sitting close to a person on the sofa or touching their shoulder as you walk by. For a "*Physical Touch* person," touch sends the clearest "I love you" message. For these people, a slap or any kind of abuse or neglect can cause extreme emotional pain.

These "languages" all sound like wonderful ways to say, "I love you," right? But there's a problem. Husbands and wives, parents and children, and even two best friends rarely speak the same love language. We all naturally reach out to other people using our own language—the one that makes us feel loved—instead of speaking the other person's language—the one that makes *them* feel loved. So even when both people go to extraordinary lengths to express love to the other, if they are each speaking their own language instead of the other person's, neither of them will feel loved.

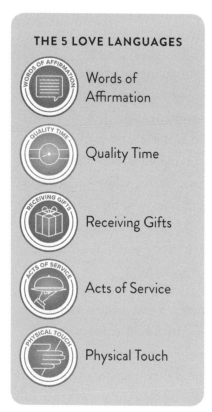

THE 5 LOVE LANGUAGES

Words of Affirmation

Quality Time

Receiving Gifts

Acts of Service

Physical Touch

Happily, there is a solution, which is the key message of the love languages books. Once people gain an understanding of the five love languages, and discover which one means the most to the significant people in their lives, they must make an effort to speak to each person in *that person's* own love language. When two people mutually embrace this idea and communicate love to each other in the way that is the most meaningful to the other person, both people feel emotionally loved. Intentional love, spoken consistently, fluently, and in the right language, deepens a relationship and equips it to weather the storms of life that will inevitably come.

THE LOVE LANGUAGES AND ALZHEIMER'S DISEASE

Wherever the five love languages have been embraced across the United States and around the world, they have revitalized relationships and pulled marriages back from the brink of divorce. Can they also help individuals, couples, and families cope with the devastating diagnosis of Alzheimer's disease? Our answer is an unequivocal *yes* and this is, in fact, the premise of our book. We believe that the love languages are tools for gently lifting a corner of the dark curtain of dementia, making it possible to sustain an emotional connection with a memory-impaired person. This is a novel idea because the love languages have been successfully utilized almost exclusively in relationships with people who are on equal footing in terms of their ability to both give and receive love. In relationships involving AD, as the disease slowly steals cognition, equal footing is first impaired and ultimately lost. Much of the relational trauma that occurs with AD happens because the person with the disease loses the ability to manage his or her side of the relationship, forcing the emotional connection into choppy and uncharted waters.

> The deep human need for love does not disappear with a diagnosis of dementia.

41

Yet, while Alzheimer's disease erases memories by literally erasing brain cells, even AD cannot erase the existence of what Gary calls the "love tank"—metaphorically, an emotional tank waiting to be filled with love. Truly, the deep human need for love does not disappear with a diagnosis of dementia. It remains ingrained in us for as long as we live.

The impact of the love languages is due, in part, to the amygdala, a brain structure not immediately affected by the disease. The amygdala is the emotion center of the brain and plays a key role in emotional memory. It prioritizes our most emotional experiences, assigning them to long-term memory where they are retained. It also helps us discern whether to consider something "good" or "bad." According to the Alzheimer's Society, the amygdala enables a person with Alzheimer's to still "recall emotional aspects of something even if they don't recall the factual content." In other words, the feeling of being loved can persist even after the actions or words that delivered the love message are forgotten.[5]

Even in late AD, when the amygdala may be affected by the disease, it is our belief that the love languages still "get through." Just because a person can no longer speak or take initiative does not mean that they no longer perceive love or know when they are being treated with kindness. Despite their difficulty in connecting thoughts, people with dementia are still able to feel deeply. Troy, a care partner for his wife, Danielle, now in late-stage AD, is keenly aware of this. He told us, "She can't do anything. She doesn't speak much anymore. She needs help with eating and bathing; she is incontinent—all the symptoms if you look at the symptom chart." Yet Troy takes every opportunity to express his love for Danielle, using all five of the love languages. He does this, not only because he truly does love her, but also because he is convinced that "no matter what goes on in the human brain, there's a core—something—that allows them to feel love. It's there in their being. They feel it; they just don't know how to say it."

Though Danielle rarely speaks, she does sometimes respond in tiny ways. "Sweet moments," said Troy, "when she still can recognize me and show me in that big ol' smile and that little laugh that she tries to do now.

"The other day we were lying on the bed watching TV and it was all quiet. Out of the blue, she just rolled over and she kissed me on my head, and I said, 'Aww, Honey, thank you!' and when I looked at her, she had a little tear in her eye."

Small responses such as this are precious evidence to Troy that Danielle does indeed feel his intentional expressions of love.

Our interactions with care partners and individuals with AD have similarly convinced us that the ability to receive emotional love endures far longer than the ability to express it, probably, for most, to the very end of the Alzheimer's journey. This makes it possible to sustain an emotional connection even with someone in the latter stages of AD. We hasten to add, however, that this kind of emotional connection is unlike any other that bonds people in love relationships. It occurs in the relational paradigm of unequal footing described above. As such, the depth and breadth of the connection lies almost entirely in the hands of the care partner.

As we write these words, like Danielle, Rebecca Shaw is nearing the end of her journey with Alzheimer's disease. Despite this, like Troy, Ed said, "Rebecca and I have been able

> The ability to receive emotional love endures far longer than the ability to express it.

to maintain emotional intimacy."

He explained, "Though there are forces that are unraveling the tapestry, you don't have to lose that person. You can maintain a really meaningful relationship with your wife or husband, mom or dad, but it is going to be *different*. You're going to find meaning in *different* ways."

He emphasizes that maintaining this kind of relational intimacy "is both intentional and sacrificial." That is, it will not happen automatically; it requires the care partner to repeatedly make "love by choice" decisions that exceed what is required in relationships unaffected by AD.

STIGMA AND DISCONNECTION

In 21st century American culture, there is still a widespread social stigma attached to diseases that affect the mind. Many people react to mental illnesses such as bipolar disorder or schizophrenia with fear, distancing themselves from the affected person. Although diagnostic codes now exist for Alzheimer's disease and other types of dementia ("neurocognitive disorder" codes), in our judgment dementia differs from mental illnesses such as depression or anxiety, which can be treated and often effectively cured with medications and/or counseling. By contrast, AD is a medical illness for which, unfortunately, there is at present no cure. However, because AD so often does "look like" a mental illness, some traditional ethnic cultures believe it is a punishment for sin and/or a social embarrassment that brings great shame upon the family.

In his past work as a radiation oncologist treating brain cancer patients, Ed observed that young children from all cultures generally tend to be fearful and standoffish toward a parent or grandparent who has cancer. The children seem to believe that if they touch Mom or Dad or their grandparent, they will "catch" their cancer. In a similar way, but on an emotional level, often when one spouse is diagnosed with AD, the other spouse, whether deliberately or unconsciously, begins to emotionally pull away from their "not well" partner. The unaffected spouse may only need some time and emotional space in which to "wrap their head around" the "A word" (Alzheimer's) and the "D word" (dementia) and what this egregious diagnosis means. Sometimes they are already grieving the losses they anticipate and fear. They may also be deeply reacting to the stigma that they personally associate with dementia. To all of this, add the stigmatizing influence of *ageism*—our youth-obsessed American cultural practice of marginalizing older people.

For any or all of these or other reasons, most unaffected spouses grow increasingly uncomfortable interacting with their newly diagnosed partner. In addition, there is a highly significant confounding factor: the person with dementia (PWD) may already have been pulling away from their spouse prior to the diagnosis, but for entirely different reasons.

As the disease begins to affect the frontal lobes of the brain, which govern personality, emotion, and social interaction, people with dementia gradually become apathetic, losing initiative, motivation, and the desire to emotionally connect with others. This apathy is global in nature and not solely directed toward their marriage partner. Their apathy is a consequence of the disease, not an indication of a lack of love for their spouse. So, as the healthy spouse is emotionally disconnecting to cope and grieve, the affected spouse is disconnecting due to the disease itself. Thus, the emotional connection is gradually untethered from both ends of the relationship. The net result over time is relational distance.

This is where Malik and Aisha found themselves. Aisha's diagnosis, Ed recalled, "just pushed them apart like two magnets of the same polarity." They were emotionally disconnected, not communicating, and had not been sexually intimate with one another for years. For both Malik and Aisha, the lack of emotional connection between them had become extremely painful. It was this emotional pain that finally compelled them to seek counseling. To use the metaphor at the beginning of the chapter, the tapestry of Malik and Aisha's marriage had begun to seriously unravel.

The emotional estrangement that this couple was experiencing, said Ed, "is the most common issue that I've encountered with couples dealing with Alzheimer's disease." In fact, he said, it's actually *typical*: "One hundred percent of the couples I have ever seen for dementia counseling have been emotionally disconnected from each other at some level." What's more, the disconnecting effects of dementia are not limited to husbands and wives. Adult children, extended family members, and friends also often pull away from the individual with dementia as well as their spouse or care partner.

"Often," Ed said, "you'll hear, 'I really learned who my friends were when I got this diagnosis.' This is true for any medical or mental health disorder. Some friends really are

> "One hundred percent of the couples I have ever seen for dementia counseling have been emotionally disconnected from each other at some level."
>
> –ED SHAW

supportive of you, people you didn't expect, and then you have others you thought were your closest friends who just fade into the sunset. Many times, what makes a person pull away from the friendship is something counselors call *transference*. Even though the disease is happening to someone else, they think, 'What if this happened to me?' and the pain of that thought pushes them away from the person with the disease. Older adults are especially fearful of AD. A 2015 study[6] published in the *Journal of Alzheimer's Disease and Other Dementias* found that 'fear of AD among older persons is greater than fear of cancer.'"

Ed said, "When a parent is diagnosed, if adult children just Google 'Alzheimer's disease risk factors,' and follow the link to the Alzheimer's Association risk factors web page, they will read, 'Those who have a parent, brother, sister or child with Alzheimer's are more likely to develop the disease.' They may panic at the words 'more likely' and not read any further. So, one of the things that complicates the parent-child relationship is that the kids are worried they are going to get it. They wonder, 'Is this going to be me in 30 years?' This has the natural effect of pushing them away from that parent because the less time they are present with the parent, the less they think about it. The busier they are with life, the less they have to confront the possibility that they might get AD. Sometimes it is intentional, but sometimes it is really unintentional. If they are just so uncomfortable with the idea of dementia in themselves or their own parent that they don't even know what to say, they will back away. So, you can see that if *Quality Time* was really important to the mother or father who had the disease, a child's backing away would be very painful for them."

Coco, whose father has AD, has not backed away from her parents, but she admits that she does worry about getting AD.

She said, "I don't want to be this kind of a burden for my husband, for my kids. I see how difficult it is emotionally, physically, and financially to have someone in this condition, and the memories that you lose. You don't have any control over it. I just hate the thought of it. So, yeah, it upsets me. I can't do anything about it, but it still lives in my thoughts."

Our friend and colleague, Dr. Julie Williams, a geriatrician with considerable expertise in dementia care, commonly observes emotional distance between AD patients and their spouses. She has noticed that the diagnosis of AD or another dementia injects "fear, pain, awkwardness, and space—emotional space" into relationships. "Sometimes it's almost cold and rigid," she said. "The patient is just sitting there, stoic and emotionally isolated, and—this is interesting—there may be an empty chair in between the patient and the spouse. There's not a lot of eye contact or communication going on verbally or nonverbally between them. I don't see a lot of hand-holding or turning to each other for support. It seems like the diagnosis of Alzheimer's disease is being borne so privately."

Dr. Williams has observed that as the disease progresses, sometimes the healthy spouse stops accompanying their husband or wife to appointments "because, mentally, they've disengaged from the relationship. They are still living in the household but they may now live in separate rooms and do separate things. It may now be an adult child who's bringing their parent in—usually a daughter who steps in and does her best to make everything okay. Most of the time, we're visiting with the caregiver child in that case." Adult children often report that their parents were not emotionally well connected before the disease occurred, said Dr. Williams, and the disease was the proverbial "straw that broke the camel's back."

Because AD so commonly unplugs the emotional connection between family members, the few strong, loving relationships she has seen really stand out to Dr. Williams. She described two couples making the Alzheimer's journey who have touched her heart.

Jane and Rick: "I will always be with you"

Jane and Rick never expected to be dealing with dementia in midlife. Barely into her 50s, Jane is already completely dependent on Rick. She has difficulty communicating and needs Rick's help with things like bathing, getting dressed, eating, and using the toilet. Rick's attitude? Dr. Williams said, "Although he is broken-hearted, he is the most loving, devoted *fan* of hers. He repeatedly refers to his wife as 'my Jane.' He says things to her like, 'Janey, we're going to get through this. We've been married 25 years and we're going to be married until we're both gone. We're going to be fine.'

"The way she responds to him is just adoring," Dr. Williams added. "She looks at him with adoring eyes. Smiling. She doesn't say much because she's losing her verbal skills, but she'll nod appropriately, usually in agreement to something positive that he's said."

As a recent visit concluded and the couple prepared to leave, Rick told Dr. Williams, "I get to have a three-hour ride with my honey at my side as we go back home." Such an expression of love, said the doctor, was "beautiful—and rare."

Ben and Sally: "Just building him up"

"This woman is fabulous," said Dr. Williams.

Sally, the wife, told her, "Ben and I love each other so much and we just always knew we were in it for the long haul. We've been hit with this terrible illness and I'm trying to understand it.

I will always love him and I will always care for him."

Dr. Williams said, "When you see them together, they are still husband and wife. She doesn't put herself in the caregiver role with him, I think as a way of preserving his dignity and his identity. You can see that she is intentionally doing that. He is her husband. He is father of the kids. She invites his partnership in making decisions. Even though his stage of disease impacts his abilities, she allows him to participate in the process. In public, she treats him as an equal."

And there's more. "She puts Ben in situations where he is valued. Walking the dog, for example. She will say, 'Thank you for walking Paddington. I don't think Paddington would go for a walk with anybody but you, Honey.' Just building him up! And she does such a good job. I could tell she was doing this for him. This is an act of kindness."

Dr. Williams recounted a conversation with the couple: She asked Ben if he had had a chance to get out and mow the lawn that summer. Ben responded, "Yeah. Yeah."

And Sally said, "Oh, Honey, tell her what you did. You went out and mowed every week and you got the yard done and it looks so nice. Dr. Williams, you should see how nice a job he does. And I never even have to ask you most of the time. You are out there and you want to get that mower started! Sometimes you're so excited that you even want to get it started without any gas in it, but by golly, one of us will manage to get gas in the mower."

Dr. Williams is quick to add that Ben is not actually capable of properly mowing a lawn. He mows across the yard in erratic patterns and tends to fixate on circling around trees, sometimes until the mower runs out of gas. Yet, she pointed out, Sally's comments are always "affirming, never critical." And, "She's usually talking *to* him, which I love. She's not speaking in the third person."

How does Ben respond to Sally?

"He smiles," Dr. Williams said. "He's rather bashful. He doesn't talk much, and that's his disease. He just watches her face. You can tell he's so focused on what she says."

Why, when most couples are disconnected by dementia, do Jane and Rick, and Sally and Ben, remain so emotionally well connected? Dr. Williams's contrasting descriptions of the patients provide the clues. In the typical disconnected couple, the person with dementia appears "emotionally isolated and very stoic" with little eye contact, little touch, and little verbal or nonverbal communication. Compare this to her description of Jane (adoring eyes . . . smiling) and her description of Ben (smiles . . . watches the face of his wife).

What makes the difference?

In Dr. Williams's and our opinion, the difference comes in the attitude of the family care partner, the main person to whom the patients are responding. Rick's loving approach to Jane, and Sally's loving approach to Ben, affirms them, preserves their dignity, and keeps the couple emotionally connected to each other. The aloof, "you-are-a-burden" approach has the opposite effect on both the patient and the relationship.

LOVE CAN CHANGE THE FUTURE

When Alzheimer's disease has driven an emotional wedge between family members or friends, the good news is that it is possible for anyone to re-establish or improve an emotional connection with a person who has AD. Troy, the loving care partner to his wife, Danielle, mentioned above, is living proof of this.

Years before Danielle was diagnosed with AD, her personality began to change. Formerly good-natured, Danielle grew increasingly argumentative, reclusive, and paranoid, behaviors that exasperated and alienated Troy. Finally, he moved out of their home. Later on, when the diagnosis of AD explained the rift between them, he returned to Danielle. His decision to return, along with the choice to begin to love her very intentionally, changed the course and tone of their relationship. Today Troy says, "I love the emotional connection and contact Danielle and I have. I just take in those moments when I can love on her. I'm going to love her as long as I've got her."

LOVE: IT'S GOOD FOR YOU

The type of positive, loving relationship that Troy, Rick, and Sally have created with their spouses benefits both the care partner and the person with AD. Connecting relationally and creating happiness for another person literally reduces stress, brain inflammation, and body inflammation for *both* people. In the absence of a positive connection, the disease can progress more rapidly and people don't live as long.

In an article reporting research published in the *Journal of the International Neuropsychological Society,* *Time* magazine reporter Maia Szalavitz wrote,[7]

"Previous studies have found that severe social isolation is at least as deadly as smoking—doubling your risk of early death—and that those with more and higher-quality relationships are at lower risk for a host of illnesses including heart disease and stroke. In fact, having strong friendships or family connections reduces your risk of early death more than exercising or avoiding obesity does—and as a bonus for most of us, it's more fun and takes less willpower.

"So why is interaction with friends and family so healing? Our stress response is intimately linked with our social connections—that's why holding Mom's hand, even as an adult, can lower blood pressure for most people, and why infants raised with minimal human contact are at many times the risk of childhood death as those with loving families. Lack of social contact is stressful for all social animals, and high chronic stress increases risk of cardiovascular disease, some cancers, obesity, all mental illnesses and addictions."

Her article focused on a research study that followed 1,138 people with no initial signs of dementia for 12 years. The study found that "the most social seniors had a 70% reduction in the rate of cognitive decline, compared with their least social peers."

Other research studies have highlighted the relationship between cognitive status, quality of life, and one's emotional connection with others. Two examples:

Reporting at the 2015 Alzheimer's Association International Conference, Dr. Nancy J. Donovan said that the US Health and Retirement Study "found that lonely people decline cognitively at a faster rate than people who report more satisfying social networks and connections." Over the study's 12-year follow-up period, the loneliest subjects experienced cognitive decline around 20% faster than participants who did not report loneliness.[8]

A 2014 study concluded that, "Feeling lonely rather than being alone is associated with an increased risk of clinical dementia in later life and can be considered a major risk factor . . ."[9]

From a strictly neuroscientific perspective, the importance of relational intimacy between dementia patients and care partners may boil down to four natural "happy chemicals" that the brain makes in response to social connection.[10] Endorphins are released when we laugh. Serotonin levels increase when a person feels significant or important, so not surprisingly, one of the hallmarks of depression is an absence of serotonin. Oxytocin is produced when we are hugged and when we receive a gift (two of the love languages—*Physical Touch* and *Gifts*—it should be noted!). Dopamine rewards and reinforces all of these pleasurable behaviors, encouraging us to repeat them.

LOVING BY CHOICE

In his counseling practice with families on the dementia journey, Ed has found the five love languages to be effective tools for reviving emotional intimacy in unraveling relationships. He often helps estranged family members bridge the gap by giving them practical homework assignments involving the love languages. When one partner is starved for touch, for example, the first step toward reconnection may be an assignment as simple as "watch a movie together and hold hands."

But, you may wonder, when dementia has already severed emotional ties, isn't it hypocritical to start expressing love to a person for whom one feels little or no love? When a woman asked Gary this very question, his response, found in *The 5 Love Languages*® chapter "Loving the Unlovely," was:

"Perhaps it would be helpful for us to distinguish between love as a feeling and love as an action. If you claim to have feelings that you do not have, that is hypocritical and such false communication is not the way to build intimate relationships. But if you express an act of love that is designed for the other person's benefit or pleasure, it is simply a choice. You are not claiming that the action grows out of a deep emotional bonding. You are simply choosing to do something for his benefit."[11] This is *hesed,* the choice-driven, sacrificial expression of love.

No matter where you and your family are on the Alzheimer's journey, and no matter how unraveled your tapestry of relationships may be, we encourage you to learn more about the five love languages. The love languages are simple tools that can be used to facilitate emotional connection in relationships complicated by dementia. The American Geriatrics Society, the American Psychiatric Society, and the American Association for Geriatric Psychiatry recommend non-pharmacological interventions as first-line treatments for the behavioral and psychiatric symptoms of dementia.[12, 13] (Non-pharmacological treatments are those that do not involve medicines.) We also see the five love languages as simple non-pharmacological interventions that can be used by anyone who cares for a person with dementia. These "love tools" can help soothe unexpressed, unmet emotional needs that can be instigators of behavioral problems in dementia patients.

You will benefit most from the chapters ahead if you know your own primary love language and the probable primary love language of the person for whom you provide care. On the concluding pages of this chapter, you will find assessment quizzes for determining these. We suggest taking these quizzes before moving on to the next chapter. Note the special instructions on the last page for determining the love language of a person in mid- to late-stage AD.

WHAT'S YOUR LOVE LANGUAGE?

Diagnostic Quizzes for Care Partners, People with Mild Cognitive Impairment (MCI), and Early- to Middle-Stage Alzheimer's Disease

Care Partners

If you are a care partner, you can discover your primary love language by completing one of the quizzes in this section. Two versions are provided: one for married people and one for singles. These are the same quizzes that appear in *The 5 Love Languages* books and on online at *5lovelanguages.com/profile*. They are also available as smartphone apps for IOS or Android.

If you are married to a person in the early stages of Alzheimer's disease, the "couples" version of the quiz is appropriate for you. If you are married to a person in the middle or late stage of AD, you may wish to take the "singles" version of the quiz. We offer this option because in advanced AD, married people often feel increasingly "single" as their partner becomes less and less capable of initiating and responding to gestures of love. If you are the adult child of a parent with AD, take the couples or singles version as appropriate.

Those with mild cognitive impairment can usually self-assess by completing the version of the profile that corresponds to their marital status.

Early- and middle-stage Alzheimer's disease

People in the early and middle stages of AD may have difficulty completing a quiz by themselves. Care partners can administer the appropriate version of the quiz to them as a one-on-one interview. Read the questions out loud, discuss the answer options, then record the person's answers.

Late middle-stage and late-stage Alzheimer's disease

See page 65.

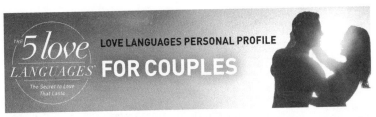

LOVE LANGUAGES PERSONAL PROFILE

FOR COUPLES

Below you will see 30 paired statements. Please circle the letter next to the statement that best defines what is most meaningful to you in your relationship. Both statements may (or may not) sound like they fit your situation, but please choose the statement that captures the essence of what is most meaningful to you, the majority of the time. Allow 10 to 15 minutes to complete the profile. Take it when you are relaxed, and try not to rush through it. If you prefer to use the free interactive version of this profile online, please visit 5lovelanguages.com.

It's more meaningful to me when . . .

1
I receive a loving note/text/email for no special reason from my loved one.	A
my partner and I hug.	E

2
I can spend alone time with my partner—just the two of us.	B
my partner does something practical to help me out.	D

3
my partner gives me a little gift as a token of our love for each other.	C
I get to spend uninterrupted leisure time with my partner.	B

4
my partner unexpectedly does something for me like filling my car with gas or doing the laundry.	D
my partner and I touch.	E

5
my partner puts his/her arm around me when we're in public.	E
my partner surprises me with a gift.	C

6
I'm around my partner, even if we're not really doing anything.	B
I hold hands with my partner.	E

7   my partner gives me a gift.   **C**

    I hear "I love you" from my partner.   **A**

8   I sit close to my partner.   **E**

    I am complimented by my loved one for no apparent reason.   **A**

9   I get the chance to just "hang out" with my partner.   **B**

    I unexpectedly get small gifts from my partner.   **C**

10   I hear my partner tell me, "I'm proud of you."   **A**

    my partner helps me with a task.   **D**

11   I get to do things with my partner.   **B**

    I hear supportive words from my partner.   **A**

12   my partner does things for me instead of just talking about doing nice things.   **D**

    I feel connected to my partner through a hug.   **E**

13   I hear praise from my partner.   **A**

    my partner gives me something that shows he/she was really thinking about me.   **C**

14   I'm able to just be around my partner.   **B**

    I get a back rub or massage from my partner.   **E**

15   my partner reacts positively to something I've accomplished.   **A**

    my partner does something for me that I know she doesn't particularly enjoy.   **D**

16   my partner and I kiss frequently.   **E**

    I sense my partner is showing interest in the things I care about.   **B**

17   my partner works on special projects with me that I have to complete.   **D**

    my partner gives me an exciting gift.   **C**

18

I'm complimented by my partner on my appearance. **A**

my partner takes the time to listen to me and really understand my feelings. **B**

19

my partner and I share nonsexual touch in public. **E**

my partner offers to run errands for me. **D**

20

my partner does a bit more than his/her normal share of the responsibilities we share (around the house, work-related, etc.). **D**

I get a gift that I know my partner put thought into choosing. **C**

21

my partner doesn't check his/her phone while we're talking. **B**

my partner goes out of their way to do something that relieves pressure on me. **D**

22

I can look forward to a holiday because of a gift I anticipate receiving. **C**

I hear the words "I appreciate you" from my partner. **A**

23

my partner brings me a little gift after he/she has been traveling without me. **C**

my partner takes care of something I'm responsible to do but I feel too stressed to do at the time. **D**

24

my partner doesn't interrupt me while I'm talking. **B**

gift giving is an important part of our relationship. **C**

25

my partner helps me out when he/she knows I'm already tired. **D**

I get to go somewhere while spending time with my partner. **B**

26

my partner and I are physically intimate. **E**

my partner gives me a little gift that he/she picked up in the course of her normal day. **C**

27

my partner says something encouraging to me. **A**

I get to spend time in a shared activity or hobby with my partner. **B**

28	my partner surprises me with a small token of her appreciation.	C
	my partner and I touch a lot during the normal course of the day.	E
29	my partner helps me out—especially if I know they're already busy.	D
	I hear my partner specifically tell me, "I appreciate you."	A
30	my partner and I embrace after we've been apart for a while.	E
	I hear my partner say how much I mean to him/her.	A

Now go back and count the number of times you circled each individual letter and write that number in the appropriate blank below.

RESULTS

A: _____ WORDS OF AFFIRMATION

B: _____ QUALITY TIME

C: _____ RECEIVING GIFTS

D: _____ ACTS OF SERVICE

E: _____ PHYSICAL TOUCH

Which love language received the highest score? This is your primary love language. If point totals for two love languages are equal, you are "bilingual" and have two primary love languages. And, if you have a secondary love language, or one that is close in score to your primary love language, this means that both expressions of love are important to you. The highest possible score for any single love language is 12.

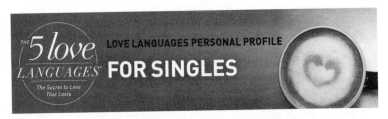

Below you will see 30 paired statements. Please circle the letter next to the statement that best defines what is most meaningful to you in your relationship. Both statements may (or may not) sound like they fit your situation, but please choose the statement that captures the essence of what is most meaningful to you, the majority of the time. Allow 10 to 15 minutes to complete the profile. Take it when you are relaxed, and try not to rush through it.

It's more meaningful to me when...

1
someone I love sends me a loving note/text/email for no special reason. **A**

I hug someone I love. **E**

2
I can spend alone time with someone I love—just us. **B**

someone I love does something practical to help me out. **D**

3
someone I love gives me a little gift as a token of our love and concern for each other. **C**

I get to spend uninterrupted leisure time with those I love. **B**

4
someone I love does something unexpected for me to help me with a project. **D**

I can share an innocent touch with someone I love. **E**

5
someone I love puts their arm around me in public. **E**

someone I love surprises me with a gift. **C**

6
I'm around someone I love, even if we're not really doing anything. **B**

I can be comfortable holding hands, high-fiving, or putting my arm around someone I love. **E**

7 I receive a gift from someone I love.   C

   I hear from someone I love that they love me.   A

8 I sit close to someone I love.   E

   I am complimented by someone I love for no apparent reason.   A

9 I get the chance to just "hang out" with someone I love.   B

   I unexpectedly get small gifts from someone I love.   C

10 I hear someone I love tell me, "I'm proud of you."   A

   someone I love helps me with a task.   D

11 I get to do things with someone I love.   B

   I hear supportive words from someone I love.   A

12 someone I love does things for me instead of just talking about doing nice things.   D

   I feel connected to someone I love through a hug.   E

13 I hear praise from someone I love.   A

   someone I love gives me something that shows they were really thinking about me.   C

14 I'm able to just be around someone I love.   B

   I get a back rub from someone I love.   E

15 someone I love reacts positively to something I've accomplished.   A

   someone I love does something for me that I know they don't particularly enjoy.   D

16 I'm able to be in close physical proximity to someone I love.   E

   I sense someone I love showing interest in the things I care about.   B

17
someone I love works on special projects with me that I have to complete.   **D**

someone I love gives me an exciting gift.   **C**

18
I'm complimented by someone I love on my appearance.   **A**

someone I love takes the time to listen to me and really understand my feelings.   **B**

19
I can share a meaningful touch in public with someone I love.   **E**

someone I love offers to run errands for me.   **D**

20
someone I love does something special for me to help me out.   **D**

I get a gift that someone I love put thought into choosing.   **C**

21
someone I love doesn't check their phone while we're talking with each other.   **B**

someone I love goes out of their way to do something that relieves pressure on me.   **D**

22
I can look forward to a holiday because I'll probably get a gift from someone I love.   **C**

I hear the words, "I appreciate you" from someone I love.   **A**

23
someone I love and haven't seen in a while thinks enough of me to give me a little gift.   **C**

someone I love takes care of something I'm responsible to do that I feel too stressed to do at the time.   **D**

24
someone I love doesn't interrupt me while I'm talking.   **B**

gift giving is an important part of the relationship with someone I love.   **C**

25
someone I love helps me out when they know I'm already tired.   **D**

I get to go somewhere while spending time with someone I love.   **B**

26 someone I love touches my arm or shoulder to show their care or concern.   E

someone I love gives me a little gift that they picked up in the course of their normal day.   C

27 someone I love says something encouraging to me.   A

I get to spend time in a shared activity or hobby with someone I love.   B

28 someone I love surprises me with a small token of their appreciation.   C

I'm touching someone I love frequently to express our friendship.   E

29 someone I love helps me out—especially if I know they're already busy.   D

I hear someone I love tell me that they appreciate me.   A

30 I get a hug from someone whom I haven't seen in a while.   E

I hear someone I love tell me how much I mean to him/her.   A

Now go back and count the number of times you circled each individual letter and write that number in the appropriate blank below.

RESULTS

A: _____ WORDS OF AFFIRMATION

B: _____ QUALITY TIME

C: _____ RECEIVING GIFTS

D: _____ ACTS OF SERVICE

E: _____ PHYSICAL TOUCH

Which love language received the highest score? This is your primary love language. If point totals for two love languages are equal, you are "bilingual" and have two primary love languages. And, if you have a secondary love language, or one that is close in score to your primary love language, this means that both expressions of love are important to you. The highest possible score for any single love language is 12.

DETERMINING THE LOVE LANGUAGE OF A PERSON WITH LATE MIDDLE-STAGE OR LATE-STAGE ALZHEIMER'S DISEASE

While there is value in knowing a person's primary pre-dementia love language, keep in mind that during late middle-stage and late-stage Alzheimer's disease, a person's love language may change. Therefore, after the midpoint of the disease, we recommend expressing love to persons with dementia using all five love languages. (We will share more about this in chapter 4, "Every Day Is the Best Day.")

If you do not know the natural pre-dementia love language of a person in late middle- or late-stage AD, but would like to make an "educated guess" about it, you may be able to deduce it through a two-step process:

Step One. Take the love languages quiz a second time on behalf of the person for whom you provide care, answering the questions the way you think he or she would have answered them before dementia.

Step Two. Answer the three questions below, which have been adapted from *The 5 Love Languages*® book:

1. Before dementia, how did your loved one most often express love to you and others?

People naturally tend to express love to others in the way that is most meaningful to them. If they regularly did acts of service for others, this may have been their own love language. If they consistently affirmed people verbally, then *Words of Affirmation* was likely their love language.

2. Before dementia, what did your loved one complain about most often?

If you or a family member went on a trip and came back empty-handed, did your loved one protest, "You didn't bring me anything"? If so, *Gifts* may have been their main love language. If he or she complained, "We don't ever spend time together," their love language was probably *Quality Time*. Says Gary, "Your complaints reveal your inner desires."

3. Before dementia, what requests did your loved one make most often?

If they asked, "Will you give me a back rub?" they were asking for physical touch. If they asked, "Would it be possible for you to clean out your closet this afternoon?" they were expressing their desire for an act of service.

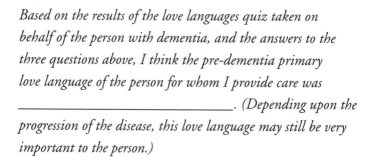

Based on the results of the love languages quiz taken on behalf of the person with dementia, and the answers to the three questions above, I think the pre-dementia primary love language of the person for whom I provide care was

_____. (Depending upon the progression of the disease, this love language may still be very important to the person.)

3

Alzheimer's Disease Puts Love to the Test

"All the book knowledge in the world cannot replace the experience of living with this."
—ABIGAIL, care partner for her mother
with Alzheimer's disease

WHY DO MOST MARRIAGES and other caring connections fray when Alzheimer's disease invades a relationship? Our deep empathy for all those touched by this disease compels us to answer, *because the journey is so hard!* We know this, not only from our own emotionally moving observations, and in Ed's case, from personal experience, but also because care partners like Troy have told us so. "This is a progressive disease and nothing gets better," he said. "Every day is harder and more emotional than the last. Short of unfaithfulness, there is probably no stronger test of marital love than Alzheimer's disease." While we so strongly encourage "love by choice" in every context of care partnering, knowing it is entirely possible, we also acknowledge that AD complicates love relationships in some very problematic, and seemingly insurmountable, ways.

"Short of unfaithfulness, there is probably no stronger test of marital love than Alzheimer's disease."—TROY

As noted earlier, the key factors in sustaining a loving connection with a person with dementia (PWD) are the outlook and efforts of the care partner. However, when the heavy load of caregiving has depleted care partners emotionally, physically, and spiritually, it becomes extremely difficult for them to summon the energy to power the intentional gestures of love we advocate. That is to say, the stress and exhaustion of caregiving can weaken or destroy the "emotional glue" that bonds the care partner to the person with dementia. For many care partners, this bond has worn so thin that just getting through the "36-hour day" takes all the energy they can muster. Most care partners, to use Gary's metaphor, have an *empty emotional tank.*

The solution—one which helps preserve the "emotional glue"—is for family members and friends to continually fill the care partner's emotional tank with intentional outpourings of love. Before we apply the five love languages specifically to care partners, it will be helpful to first highlight seven aspects of Alzheimer's disease that, in our opinion, most threaten the fragile emotional bonds of relationships.

SEVEN THREATS TO THE "EMOTIONAL GLUE"

The Delusion of Infidelity

A delusion is the belief that something is true when it is not. Delusions can occur when a person has misinterpreted sensory input—what is seen, heard, or felt. Memory loss, declining visual and spatial function, and other cognitive changes can play a role too. About 70 percent of people with AD will have delusional thoughts at some point.[1] While delusions can be present early in the disease, they usually occur later due to brain changes that typically begin in the middle stage. Sometimes delusions are triggered by sensory overload: bright lights, too much noise, or shadows that distort the appearance of common objects. As a result, people, objects, and situations that were once familiar may now seem confusing or threatening. Common delusions are believing that a stranger has been in the house, or that people on TV are actually present in the room. Some people believe that their real spouse, adult child, or even a pet or their house has been replaced by a lookalike imposter, a delusion known as Capgras syndrome.

Sometimes people have paranoid delusions. These are false beliefs that make the person suspicious or distrustful. A person may believe, for example, that someone is spying on her. Someone may complain that their money, clothes, or other possessions are being stolen. Paranoid beliefs usually affect behavior. People may respond to the belief that their possessions are being stolen by accusing family members of theft. They may also begin hiding or hoarding things. Care partners have told us of loved ones hoarding everything from candy to golf balls! Of course, it is always possible that someone's complaint is actually true, so it is wise to investigate before assuming it is delusional.

Of all the common paranoid delusions, none is likely to place more stress on a marriage than the false belief that one's spouse is having an affair. In this scenario, the person with AD becomes convinced of their spouse's infidelity despite the lack of any evidence. Because delusions seem so real to the person experiencing them, no amount of reasoning or explaining will convince the person of their spouse's faithfulness. The tears and emotional angst stirred by accusations of infidelity are painful and disruptive to any marriage, and marriages involving dementia are no exception. (In chapter 5 we share a strategy for dealing with delusions and other challenging behaviors.)

Mistaken Identity

When AD affects not only memory but also the parts of the brain that allow us to recognize faces and interpret sensory input, a person may become confused about the identity of family members or others they have known for years. The experience Ed described in the first chapter, when his wife no longer recognized him as her husband, is an example of this. For Ed, you may recall, this was an emotionally painful experience.

Sarah's experience was similar. "It was the first thing that really crushed me," she said.

"One day my husband, Bob, introduced me to a lady as his sister. He said, 'Have you ever met my sister, Lucy?' And my mouth just dropped! Later that same day he turned to our son-in-law and said, 'Have you ever met my sister, Lucy?'

"This really upset me at the time. That was two years ago and I think for a long time he thought I *was* Lucy. Bob actually has a sister named Lucy. He knows I'm his wife now, but he thinks that he's only visiting me."

After surviving the initial shock, Sarah and Ed learned to remind themselves that their mate's confusion about their identity is due to the disease. In families where there has been no diagnosis of AD or a diagnosis but little education about the disease, the mistaken identity experience may be, as it was for Sarah, crushing, with no information to help mitigate the emotional sting.

Odd Behavior

Every dementia care partner would do well to memorize this sentence from *The 36-Hour Day*: "When a person does something odd or inexplicable, it is usually because some part of the brain has failed to do its job."[2] Care partners have told us many stories of "odd or inexplicable" behavior by their loved ones:

- Sam's wife is obsessed with watering their indoor plants. She waters them daily and the plants are drowning. One day when the water started to overflow the pots, Sam cried, "Stop! Stop!" but his wife wouldn't stop. They argued about it for a few minutes before Sam gave up. He decided to put plastic bags underneath the pots to catch the overflow.

- Abigail's mom got up at 2 a.m. and got dressed. She said she was waiting for her ride. When Abigail told her that no one was coming to pick her up in the middle of the night, Abigail said, "She looked at me like I was crazy."

- Marcy brought her uncle, Jerry, to her home to give his care partner a break. Marcy was making cookies as a treat for Jerry. While the cookies were baking, she showed Jerry the sand dollars she had brought back from her beach trip. Jerry was closely examining a sand dollar in his hand when the oven timer buzzed. Marcy walked across the kitchen, opened the oven, and pulled the cookie sheets out. As the delicious aroma of freshly baked cookies wafted over the room, Marcy heard a loud *crunch* . . .

- Paul asked his wife for a bowl of snowflakes. She knew he meant ice cream.

- Bob thought that he and his wife, Sarah, were going on a trip so he could take a new job. He filled the trunk of their car with a miter saw, levels, hammers, and an assortment of other tools. When Bob was busy doing something else, Sarah unloaded the trunk and brought all the tools back inside. Bob carried the tools outside again and reloaded the trunk. Sarah patiently unloaded them again. The loading and unloading went on for over a week.

Loss of Sexual Intimacy

One of the least talked about aspects of Alzheimer's disease is the fact that it eventually robs a couple of their sexual relationship. The majority of senior adults remain sexually active well into their 80s, and in early AD people can still continue to enjoy sexual activity. As time goes on, however, numerous factors eventually conspire to sabotage sexual intimacy.

As the disease invades the brain's frontal lobes, people with AD slowly lose the ability to initiate anything, including sexual activity. In addition, as memory fades, people literally forget how to make love. When they can no longer remember their former foreplay

> When a person with AD no longer recognizes their spouse, most care partners feel uncomfortable about continuing the sexual relationship.

"routine," people with AD may feel too embarrassed or inadequate to engage in sexual activity. Some people also become hypersensitive to touch and thus averse to sexual activity.

As in Ed's story, when a person with AD no longer recognizes their spouse, or as in Sarah's story, when the spouse is mistaken for another relative, most care partners feel uncomfortable about continuing the sexual relationship. Also, as noted previously, even when intimacy is not hindered by the disease itself, the emotional gulf between the couple often nullifies the desire for physical intimacy.

Some spouses tell us they don't want the sexual part of their relationship back. Pam says that for her, it's because her husband doesn't want to shower and because his bathroom habits are "off-putting." Most husbands and wives, however, say they miss sexual intimacy with their spouse.

Disinhibition

When the frontal lobes of the brain are affected by dementia, people have less control over their "manners" and socially appropriate behaviors. This reduced ability to control impulses is called *disinhibition*. Disinhibited behaviors include swearing, showing no empathy, shoplifting, rudeness, insensitivity, interacting poorly with others, and, infrequently, masturbation, public urination, or disrobing in public. About 36 percent of those with AD will exhibit some sort of disinhibition during the course of their disease.[3] Disinhibition is much more common among those with frontotemporal dementia (FTD).

Disinhibition can extend to sexual behaviors. As mentioned above, most people with AD grow apathetic about sex; but with more frontal lobe involvement, according to Dr. Julie Williams, "you may end up getting more disinhibition." When sexually disinhibited behaviors are focused on one's spouse, the PWD may be insensitive, aggressive, and demanding, exhibiting anger if the spouse denies the advances. When sexual disinhibition is directed to people other than the spouse, it may range from off-color remarks to overt sexual advances. This is the disease at work, causing the person to be confused about the identities of others or even forgetting that he or she has a spouse. Dr. Williams says that when sexual disinhibition is directed at someone other than the person's spouse, it is emotionally challenging for the healthy spouse, who, though hurt, must "place the behavior in the context of the disease. And that's not easy."

Sarah said that when she arrived to pick up her husband from his adult daycare program, "he was holding hands with one of the women who is also a patient. I just chuckled to myself. I figured it was going to happen. I have kind of accepted it, even though it's hard to accept."

Repeating

When AD has severely eroded short-term memory, and a person simply cannot remember things from one minute to the next, conversations can get stuck in an endless loop. Ed said, "When the person with the disease keeps asking the same question or referring to an event over and over it frustrates their spouse. The spouse gets short-tempered and says, 'You've asked me that ten times! Why can't you remember that? Write it down. Here's a Post-it note. Stick this on your forehead.'" It takes a lot of patience to answer a question for the fifteenth time in as kind and neutral a way as the first time it is asked.

I (Debbie) got my first glimpse of this one day when I was

asked to sit with an Alzheimer's patient while his wife was getting information about a research study. This gentleman and I were sitting less than 10 feet from the room where his wife was. Our conversation went something like this:

"Hi Bill. I'm Debbie. I'm going to chat with you while your wife talks with the doctor."

"Okay. Where's my wife?"

I pointed to the closed door and said, "She's in that room right there talking with the doctor."

Bill picked up a magazine and started flipping through it. Then he abruptly put it down and asked, "Where's my wife?"

"See that door right there? She's in that room. She'll be out in a few minutes."

"What's she doing in there?"

"She is talking with the doctor."

Hoping to distract Bill, I asked, "How many children do you have, Bill?"

"I'm not sure. Where's my wife?"

I told him again. He picked up the same magazine, put it down, and asked, "Where's my wife?"

Shadowing

People like Bill, in the latter part of their AD journey, want to stay physically close to their primary care partner. This person, more than anyone else, makes them feel safe in an increasingly incomprehensible world. They will literally follow their care provider around the house all day long. Betsy told us that her husband, Brent, even follows her to the bathroom. "It's like being glued at the hip," she said, clearly exasperated.

Writer Carole Larken has noted, "After a while this behavior becomes disconcerting and even annoying to the Alzheimer's caregiver. The caregiver essentially loses their own personal space and begins to feel smothered by the person with dementia."[4]

CAREGIVER BURDEN

The seven aspects of AD described above, along with others not mentioned here, impose a new, *abnormal* "normal" on relationships that can skew or totally unglue them. Everyone who knows the person with AD must grapple with the fact that he or she is no longer the same spouse, parent, sibling, or friend they knew before the disease set in. While there is comfort in knowing that the person has not intentionally changed, this knowledge doesn't make daily life easier for family care providers. They carry an emotional "backpack" known in professional literature as *caregiver burden*. While the contents of care partners' backpacks differ according to their life circumstances, nearly all of them contain the weighty components of grief and stress.

Care Partner Grief

In his foreword to the book, *The Longest Loss: Alzheimer's Disease and Dementia*, Dr. Peter Rabins noted that all dementias "are associated with a grieving process in both the person with dementia and those who love and care for them."[5]

Gradually, people with AD lose the ability to do things for themselves, to relate to others, and to remember who they are. With each of these losses, family care partners lose something, too:

• The personality of the loved one that has made their relationship unique

76

- The companionship of the person, perhaps including sexual intimacy

- The help the care partner has been accustomed to receiving from him or her

- The freedom the care partner had when caregiving was a smaller part of daily life

- The future that had been planned with the loved one

Some of these losses are especially difficult because they are not as clear-cut or definitive, as when, for example, a death occurs.

Betty's husband has AD. Her friend observed, "You're married and widowed at the same time." This comment reveals the ambiguous nature of Betty's losses: though she is married, in some ways her husband's disease has rendered her single. Betty's ambiguous grief contrasts with the more concrete grief of divorce or death. If Betty were grieving a divorce, both she and her ex-husband would still be alive, but one or both of them would have chosen the divorce. If she were grieving her husband's death, only she would be alive, but neither spouse would have chosen the death. But since Betty's husband has AD, her grief is a hybrid: both she and her husband are still alive, and neither of them chose the disease.

The grief of Alzheimer's disease is intermittent. It typically surges initially at the time of diagnosis, then levels off in the middle of the disease, only to resurge again as the journey's end approaches. The course of grief changes along with the course of the disease. In the beginning, usually both the family and the PWD share the grief of the diagnosis. In the early and middle stages of the disease, loved ones and the PWD grieve different things. Loved ones grieve the diagnosed person's declining cognition, changing personality, and behaviors; the PWD grieves their loss of abilities and independence. In late AD, when the PWD has lost insight about what is happening to them, family members grieve the journey's end alone.

Care Partner Stress

According to the Alzheimer's Association, 83 percent of caregiving in the U.S. is done by unpaid family members. In 2015 about 15.7 million unpaid American care partners provided 18.1 billion hours of care to those with AD and other types of dementia.[6] Many who provide care for a family member are also holding down a job and raising children as well. In a poll of women in a dual caring role, 53 percent said that caring for a person with AD was more challenging than caring for children.[7]

Regardless of pay, training, or relationship to a PWD, caregiving is often a lonely, stressful, thankless task. Many family care partners have little or no physical help or emotional support and sometimes no one to step in and give them a much needed break. Those who are "on call" 24/7 and/or frequently sleep-deprived are often overwhelmed and living in a state of chronic, unrelieved stress. Chronic stress does more than wear us out. By increasing the presence of the stress hormones adrenaline and cortisol in the bloodstream, unrelenting stress takes a serious toll on the body. Excessive cortisol is thought to elevate blood pressure and suppress the immune system, making care partners more vulnerable to illness.

Highly stressed care partners are more likely to have a long-term health problem such as heart disease, stroke, cancer, diabetes, or arthritis. And, because they are more focused on caring for the PWD than for themselves, they are more likely to be significantly overweight and less likely to exercise or cook healthy meals.[8]

Care partner stress also takes an emotional toll. Not so surprisingly, 40 percent of family care partners suffer from clinical depression. The more severe the cognitive impairment of the person for whom they care, the more likely the care partner is to be depressed.[9] Gracie said, "I love life! I get up in the morning and open the shutters, grateful to be here, and within 30 minutes I'm reminded of where I really am. I am in the midst of dementia. And my joy so quickly fades. Every day, I deal with depression."

_____

"Divorce may cross the mind of many care partners at some point."
—DR. JULIE WILLIAMS

_____

Many care partners also struggle with anxiety and a host of emotions. We asked some of them to name the emotion that most characterizes their caregiving experience:

Cherie: sadness
Stephen: frustration
Richard: guilt
Peter: loneliness
Marsha: resentment, regret, and bitterness

Marsha explained, "This is a second marriage for me. Maybe if I had tried harder in my first marriage I wouldn't be in this situation now. I feel cheated. I want to move on with my life."

While not all care partners may admit to it, Dr. Williams told us, "Divorce may cross the mind of many care partners at some point." Ed says, "Without a doubt, the emotional toll is greater and family issues are more complex in second marriages when dementia affects one of the partners." While all of the care partners we interviewed for this book have dismissed divorce as an option for themselves, they understand the very human wish to escape an emotionally painful, physically exhausting situation.

CAREGIVER BURDEN: OUR SURVEYS

Using a self-report survey called the Zarit Caregiver Burden Interview, we polled 50 dementia care partners participating in support groups. This questionnaire asks respondents to use a five-point scale to indicate how they feel about certain aspects of caregiving. In answer to the question, *"Do you feel that because of the time you spend with your relative that you don't have enough time for yourself?"* about 80 percent said they feel this way "sometimes," "quite frequently," or "nearly always." In response to the question, *"Do you feel stressed between caring for your relative and trying to meet other responsibilities for your family or work?"* 39 out of 50 said they feel this way "sometimes," "quite frequently," or "nearly always."

We also surveyed 100 care partners using the Marwit-Meuser Caregiver Grief Inventory. This questionnaire measures worry and isolation, sadness and longing, and personal sacrifice burden. More than half agreed with the statements, *"Independence is what I've lost . . . I don't have the freedom to go and do what I want,"* and, *"I wish I had an hour or two to myself each day to pursue personal interests."*

SOCIAL SUPPORT REALLY MATTERS

As AD progresses, those affected become increasingly dependent upon the provision and mercy of their care partners. When someone is caring for a dependent individual, it creates an unequal dyad in which one person mainly gives and the other mainly receives. In such off-balance, high-stress caregiving scenarios, there is potential for abuse. According to a 2009 study reported by the National Center on Elder Abuse (NCEA), "close to 50 percent of people with dementia experience some kind of abuse."[10] In 2010, another study found that "47 percent of participants with dementia had been mistreated by their caregivers."[11]

Abuse occurs not only in worst-case scenarios involving poverty or drug addiction, but sometimes also when persons with AD are beloved family members. Even in environments where physical and financial needs are met, a dependent dyad can go horribly wrong when care partner stress is excessive, unrelenting, and unrelieved, pushing caregivers to an emotional breaking point.

High care-partner stress is also of concern for two other important reasons. First, and rather ironically, heavy caregiver burden and the unhealthy lifestyle that often accompanies caregiving can actually increase a spouse care partner's own risk for dementia. A 2010 study found that husbands and wives caring for a spouse with dementia are six times more likely to develop dementia than people whose spouses are dementia-free.[12] While many factors are associated with the onset of dementia, research has not yet shown any clear "cause and effect" relationship. One likely contributor, however, is the excessive cortisol triggered by chronic stress. This increases brain inflammation, a known accelerator of cognitive decline. Experts also think that the social isolation of caregiving, coupled with little physical activity, poor sleep, and a shift to fast food and processed foods may all contribute to care partners' increased risk for dementia.

The second reason for concern comes from the 1999 Caregiver Health Effects Study. The investigators wrote, "[Our] data indicate that caregivers who provide support to their spouse and report caregiver strain are 63% more likely to die within 4 years than non-caregivers." The study defined "strained caregivers" as those between the ages of 66 and 96 with "significantly higher levels of depressive symptoms, higher levels of anxiety, and lower levels of perceived health…much less likely to get enough rest in general, have time to rest when they are sick, or have time to exercise."[13]

Twenty-seven of the 50 care partners we surveyed with the Zarit Caregiver Burden Interview responded affirmatively to the question, *Do you feel your health has suffered because of your involvement with your relative?* Most of the care partners we interviewed one-on-one also told us that caring for their loved one had negatively impacted their health. Sarah said, "I was diagnosed with type 2 diabetes and I think it was brought on by stress. And, because I worry and take care of my husband, I forget myself."

Sandra's story in particular illustrates why care partners find it so difficult to address their own health needs.

Sandra said, "I am an eater when I get stressed. I needed to start taking care of myself because my numbers—blood pressure, cholesterol, and weight—were all too high. There were definitely signs that my health had deteriorated and it was time to own what the numbers were and manage them." She made an appointment with her doctor. She had planned to take her husband, Aaron, with her, but on the day of the appointment, he refused to get dressed. Rather than cancel the appointment, she asked a neighbor to keep an eye on Aaron.

Returning home after the appointment, she saw police cars in her neighborhood. When she walked into her house she found her husband and a policeman. She learned that the neighbor had somehow missed Aaron's escape, and that the officer had responded to a report that Aaron, wearing no clothes, had walked to a nearby school. That "disaster," said Sandra, "was my attempt at owning my health." Aaron declined rapidly after this incident and Sandra recalled, "My interest in focusing on my health was put on the back burner while we dealt with the myriad of issues that ensued."

The Alzheimer's Association notes that caring for a PWD does not always result in care partner stress or negative health consequences. In its 2015 *Facts and Figures* report, the organization states that the stress of caregiving varies according to "dementia severity, how challenging caregivers perceive certain aspects of care to be, *available social support* and caregiver personality" [emphasis added].[14] Similarly, the National Institute on Aging states that "caregivers who have *strong support systems* and well-developed coping skills may be able to weather the stresses of caring for a loved one with AD" [emphasis added].[15]

Our view, in light of these findings, is that efforts to undergird stressed-out care partners are more than mere acts of kindness. Social support is a care partner intervention that can help prevent patient abuse and reduce care partners' risk for dementia, illness, and premature death. *Social support really matters.*

THE LOVE Rx

The weight of the burdens in a care partner's "backpack" has a lot to do with how much they shoulder alone. One goal of this chapter is to encourage social support, using care partners' own love languages to reduce their caregiver burden. The five love languages can be effective tools for communicating the loving support that softens or reverses some of the harmful effects of stress. Those inside and outside of the family can use care partners' love languages to help them "carry the backpack." Whenever a care partner's emotional love tank is empty, the love languages can be creatively used to help fill it up again.

FAMILY AND FRIENDS: WAYS TO SUPPORT CARE PARTNERS

Grief expert Dr. Alan Wolfelt distinguishes between grief and mourning. Grief, he says, is internal. Mourning is external, an experience that we share with others. What often happens, he says, is that many people "end up grieving within themselves in isolation, instead of mourning outside of themselves in the presence of loving companions."[16]

In her book, *Loving Someone Who Has Dementia*, Dr. Pauline Boss tells care partners, "What you need to avoid is being isolated in a relationship that may never be reciprocal again."[17] Many care partners speak of the loneliness they experience as their loved one declines, leaving them more and more emotionally isolated. Isolation can be lethal to care partner endurance. Ed said, "Human beings are creatures of relationship. People bail out because caregiving can be very, very lonely."

> "People bail out because caregiving can be very, very lonely." —ED SHAW

Intentional expressions of love, creatively administered via the five love languages, help remedy isolation, one of the most painful aspects of care partnering. If you know a person caring for a PWD, do not underestimate the immense value of reaching out to them in love and support. This is what transforms the isolation of grief into the healing experience of mourning in community with others.

USING THE FIVE LOVE LANGUAGES TO
REACH OUT TO CARE PARTNERS

Alzheimer's care partners, like all of us, feel most emotionally loved when others speak their love language. To tailor loving outreach to an individual care partner, ask them to complete the love languages quiz (in chapter 2) so that both of you can discover their primary love language. Then, armed with this knowledge, undergird the care partner using the language that "speaks love" to them most clearly. Never lose sight of the fact that your efforts to benefit care partners ultimately help the person in their care as well.

Speaking Acts of Service

Care partners are often in need of practical help. Elderly care partners may resist help if they were raised to believe it is their spousal duty to do everything themselves. Experts say that it's easier for care partners to accept help if the offers are very specific and the person making the offer is gently persistent. Offers to help that are specific sound like this:

"I am going to the grocery store this afternoon. What can I pick up for you?"

"I'm making vegetable soup today. Is 4:00 a good time to bring some over to you?"

"I have a couple of hours free on Thursday morning. How about if I take Fred for a drive so you can have some time to yourself?"

There are endless acts of service that could be of genuine help to a care partner. Some ideas: mow their lawn, do their laundry, pick up a prescription, share veggies from your garden, shovel snow, rake leaves, make home repairs, offer to stay with the PWD so the care partner can attend a support group, run errands, exercise, nap, or go to a doctor's appointment.

Speaking Words of Affirmation

In *The 5 Love Languages*®, Gary writes, "Psychologist William James said that possibly the deepest human need is the need to feel appreciated. *Words of Affirmation* will meet that need in many individuals."[18] Research suggests that when family members show their appreciation for care partners' efforts, they perceive their burden as lighter. Ed says that whenever he talks on the phone with his daughter, Leah, she almost always tells him, "Dad, you're doing a good job." Ed has shared this simple but powerful encouragement with many of his patients and counseling clients.

Most care partners we interviewed told us they struggle with feelings of guilt—guilt because they are not doing more for the person with the disease, guilt when they take time away for themselves, or guilt because they are cognitively normal and their loved one is not. Verbal encouragement can help a weary care partner extend grace to herself, alleviating guilt, as words from others affirm how great a load she carries and how well she carries it. Care partners whose love language is *Words of Affirmation* may feel loved by phone calls, greeting cards, text messages, or emails that express admiration for the care partner's efforts. Complimenting the care partner, both privately and in the presence of others, may also be very meaningful: "Helen does an amazing job caring for John—she is so patient with him."

Another idea is to hang a cork board, chalkboard, or white board where family and friends can pin notes or write inspirational quotes or words of encouragement that the care partner will see each day. For a fun, modern twist on this idea, apply latex chalkboard paint to a wall, door, or table and keep a supply of colored chalk on hand.

Speaking Quality Time

Gary defines quality time as "giving someone your undivided attention."[19] The choice-driven, intentional love called *hesed* is "*Quality Time* love." In chapter 2 we encouraged care partners to reach into the lives of those for whom they provide care with *hesed* love. Here, we prescribe generous doses of *hesed* for the care partner.

Reaching out to care partners with *Quality Time* is the best balm we know for the isolation of caregiving. Spending quality time may mean listening to a care partner who is lonely or aching with grief. It can also mean involving him or her in pleasant experiences that provide respite and build friendship. Care partners whose love language is *Quality Time* may especially appreciate one-on-one time with a sympathetic listener who focuses on what the care partner has to say and sincerely seeks to understand what he or she is feeling. Likewise, participation in a care partner support group might be helpful. And all care partners need time away from the PWD, doing something fun with a companion.

Speaking Physical Touch

When a PWD has lost the ability to initiate affection or has become averse to touch, it leaves a void in the spouse care partner's life. Friends and family can reach out with hugs, pats, fist bumps, high-fives, or a comforting hand on the care partner's shoulder. Depending on the relationship, a foot rub or a back massage might also be appreciated.

Ed's primary love language is *Physical Touch*. His family and friends know that he is a "hugger." One of his closest male friends, Bing, is Japanese-American. Because of his culture, and also because of the way Bing is wired, he is not naturally a *Physical Touch* kind of guy. Nevertheless, Bing is intentional not only about meeting with Ed weekly for some guy time, but also about giving Ed a "man hug" when they depart. Bing recognizes the importance of *Physical Touch* to his friend, and intentionally reaches out with a hug to support Ed's caregiving of Rebecca.

If a care partner's love language is *Physical Touch,* these gestures may help to fill their emotional tank:

- When you speak with the person, occasionally touch them briefly on the shoulder or elbow (considered "safe" places to touch). If you pray at mealtimes, hold their hand as the prayer is spoken.

- Tactile experiences. Female care partners may appreciate a relaxing at-home "spa escape" while you spend time with the PWD: draw a bubble bath, light a scented candle, add soft music, and provide some soothing after-bath lotion.

- Tactile gifts. On gift-giving occasions, or for no special reason, give a cozy afghan, a pair of fuzzy slippers or gloves, a foot spa massager, an "egg crate" mattress topper, a gift certificate for a massage, or even a stuffed animal.

Speaking Gifts

As mentioned earlier, gifts can be tangible or intangible. When the intangible gift is what Gary calls "the gift of self or the gift of presence,"[20] the language of *Gifts* merges with the language of *Quality Time.* One's physical presence is itself the gift and it says, "I care about you."

Gifts that are tangible can be personal treats such as chocolates or concert tickets, or things that provide practical help.

When tangible gifts are well-chosen, the language of *Gifts* again merges with other love languages, as in the example above of giving tactile gifts to a person whose love language is *Physical Touch*. A care partner whose love language is *Gifts* may feel loved and also be helped by practical gifts such as meals that can be frozen and kept on hand, gift cards for gas, groceries, or restaurants, or hiring a house cleaning or lawn care service for the care partner. Adult children can give the gift of respite time to their caregiving parent by spending a couple of mornings a week with the PWD or hiring a professional caregiver to help with tasks like bathing and dressing.

A LANGUAGE FOR A LIFETIME

Our love language preferences are apparently "hard-wired" into our natural makeup. Gary said, "I think that our primary love language tends to stay with us for a lifetime."[21] Thus, while nothing about the caregiving experience can alter the care partner's main love language, Gary believes that circumstances can elevate the importance of another love language for a time. For example, even if *Acts of Service* is not a care partner's love language, if he is exhausted from caregiving and miserable with the flu, when a friend shows up to shovel his snowy driveway, this generous act of service may fill his emotional tank to the brim.

CULTURAL SENSITIVITY

Attitudes about caregiving and accepting help vary among cultures. While African Americans are twice as likely to develop AD as white Americans,[22] African American families utilize fewer agency services than white families.[23] Hispanic/Latino Americans,

Asian Americans, and white Americans may all have different beliefs about dementia.

As mentioned previously, some cultures believe that dementia is punishment for past sins and/or an embarrassment that brings shame upon the family. If families believe they should hide AD from outsiders, they may resist help and support. Therefore, in the interest of "cultural competence," before reaching out to a family with a cultural background that is different than yours, first research the beliefs of their culture. Specifically, it will be helpful to understand their beliefs about healthcare, dementia, and the appropriateness of accepting help from those outside the family. Often, the best way to do this is to befriend a member of the culture and ask him or her to teach you about their culture. In addition, the primary care partner for the person with AD should be asked what would be most helpful to make sure support is provided in a culturally appropriate way. Health educators use this same "key informant" approach in order to design culturally appropriate public health interventions.

SELF-CARE FOR CARE PARTNERS

The authors of *The 36-Hour Day* wrote, "The well-being of the person who has dementia depends entirely on your well-being. *It is essential that you find ways to care for yourself so that you will not exhaust your own emotional and physical resources*" [emphasis in original].[24] We agree and urge you to make your own health an even higher priority than the health of the person in your care.

Does that sound selfish?

I (Debbie) used to think so. In *A Season at Home,* a book for stay-at-home moms (now out of print), I wrote about the experience that changed my thinking. I was flying from North Carolina to Los Angeles with my two-year-old son. Perhaps I listened more attentively to the pre-flight safety speech because Chris was with me. The flight attendant explained that the oxygen masks would drop from above if cabin pressure was lost. She said, "If you are traveling with a small child, put your own oxygen mask on before attempting to assist the child." This statement bothered me. I wondered, "If Chris and I both needed oxygen, wouldn't it be selfish to take care of myself first?"

I pondered this for a while before finally deciding that the airline was right. A child might resist the parent's attempt to get the mask over the child's head. While the parent was trying to win the power struggle, he or she might pass out from lack of oxygen. Then, with no one to help, the child might pass out too. But by instructing the parent to do the "selfish" thing, the airline increases the chances that both will get oxygen.

I wrote, "The lesson I learned that day is this: it's not selfish for mothers to get their own needs met; it's smart."[25]

It's every bit as smart to think this same way when caring for a person with dementia. To be *able* to care for that person, you *must* care for yourself. To frame that another way, what would happen to the person in your care if something happened to you? Resolve to be intentional about self-care in light of these two sobering facts:

- Half of care partners report that their own declining health compromises their caregiving ability.[26]

- As noted earlier, super-stressed care partners are 63 percent more likely to die within four years than non-caregivers.[27]

CAREGIVING IS A TEAM SPORT

If you are a care partner, do not stoically try to go it alone. Part of caring for yourself is allowing yourself to receive care from others. Ed tells care partners that caregiving is a team sport. His counsel is based on the advice he was once given by Rebecca's physician, Dr. Jeff Williamson. He told Ed, "You have reached a point in this journey where you can no longer think of yourself as helping others; you must now become one who is helped." Ed now passes this same advice on to other care partners. He tells them, "If you don't involve your family and others in sharing caregiving responsibilities, you're more likely to burn out or bail out. You'll get a bad attitude if you never get a break. You have to have some time for yourself. It makes you a better care partner."

> To be *able* to care for a person with dementia, you *must* care for yourself.

Few people would dispute the wisdom of making caregiving a team sport. The problem is that most care partners don't have enough people on their team. While some people will naturally circle around an Alzheimer's patient and their care partner, most will need an invitation to join the care team. Ed suggests making a list of potential care team members. He said, "Simply share the Alzheimer's diagnosis with them. Tell them what stage the disease is in, and what kind of help you need. Be specific. For example, say, 'I really need help taking care of the lawn. Could you take over the mowing?' When the answer is 'Sorry, I don't have time,' be gracious and non-judgmental. There are lots of reasons that people don't or can't help."

Often, those who volunteer to help are people the care partner never expected to do so. Other times, as Sonya discovered, people whose support is expected pull away. When Sonya asked her two closest family members to join her team, both declined. One told her, "I have an issue with you talking about how hard this is for you when your husband is the one who is losing his life." Fortunately, when Sonya asked her closest church friends to join her team, their response was, "We have your back." She told them, "If you want to know how I am, call me; I need the human voice. Hug me; if you don't touch me, nobody does." Said Sonya, "They have just stepped up to the plate beautifully."

Just as with sports teams, not everyone can or should play the same role on the care partner support team. Some people are uncomfortable around people with AD; others are truly gifted to work with them. Some people have time and energy, but little money. Others have money, but little time and energy. Some people are natural encouragers; others are natural doers, always working in the kitchen, the yard, or on cars or computers. The point is, though people vary widely in their talents and circumstances, most everyone can contribute something to a care partner support team. They just need to be asked to help.

Many care partners benefit immensely from participating in a support group. Since members are all facing similar challenges, these groups offer a level of camaraderie that can be hard to find elsewhere. Sarah observed, "People who haven't been around Alzheimer's don't understand what you are really going through." Betsy tearfully shared with her support group something she had not shared with others because, she said, "I don't have to explain it to you all."

As "team captain," be proactive about using your own love language to take care of yourself. For example, if your love language is

Receiving Gifts, when you need an emotional boost, buy yourself a small treat such as a chocolate bar or a magazine. If you are an *"Acts of Service* person," keep a list of ways that others can help you and ask for help when you need it. If *Physical Touch* means the most to you, schedule a massage or facial. If your love language is *Words of Affirmation,* call a friend. If *Quality Time* tops your list, when someone volunteers to spend time with the person for whom you provide care, invite a friend to take a walk with you.

Your team will be better equipped to support you if they understand what means the most to you. Explain the five love languages to your team and share your primary love language with them (or give them a copy of this book or one of the *5 Love Languages®* books).

TIPS FOR CARE PARTNERS

If you are a care partner, there are many things we could suggest to maintain your health and quality of life. Here are three we believe are particularly important:

1. **Exercise.** Exercise improves the health of the brain's blood vessels, allowing better delivery of nutrients and oxygen to brain cells. In one research study, participants who exercised regularly at home showed "significant improvement" in their sense of burden and in their physical wellbeing. They did not feel as weary and had better sleep quality. Researchers speculated that "the increased physical activity . . . led to an improvement in the quality of sleep, which in turn improved physical and psychological symptoms."[28] We urge you to be physically active for at least 150 minutes a week. If you have health issues, talk to your doctor about what type of exercise is best for you.

2. **Sleep**. Six to seven hours of nightly sleep may help the brain clear away the toxic beta amyloid protein that leads to AD.[29] Adequate sleep is absolutely vital for care partners. While one of the benefits of exercise is improved sleep quality, if the person for whom you care is up and down all night, even if you exercise your sleep will suffer. This is a problem you must solve. Can you afford to hire a nighttime caregiver? If not, do you have a support team friend or family member who, if asked, would be willing to stay with the PWD each day for an hour or two so you can take a nap?

3. **Find a counselor and take an antidepressant if needed.** Ed said, "Even chronic sadness can deplete your brain's 'happy chemicals.' This is the ninth year of our Alzheimer's journey. I take antidepressants and they have been very helpful. I also have a counselor to talk to." If your quality of life is diminished by chronic sadness or depression, talk to your doctor about prescribing an antidepressant medicine and providing a referral to a mental health professional for counseling support. Also seek an AD caregiver support group.

4

Every Day Is the Best Day

"My yesterdays are disappearing, and my tomorrows
are uncertain, so what do I live for?
I live for each day. I live in the moment."
–from the movie *Still Alice*

THERE IS A POIGNANT urgency to loving someone with Alzheimer's disease. There is *urgency* because, as Troy said in the previous chapter, "This is a progressive disease and nothing gets better." This is why Ed tells care partners, "Every day is the best day." He means that because no future day with Alzheimer's is likely to be better than the one called *today*, it is important to make the most of each day. Thus, the urgency is also *poignant,* stirring the emotions.

Ed is personally acquainted with the poignant urgency. "I always envisioned Rebecca and me growing old together," he said. "But when she was diagnosed with Alzheimer's disease, being a doctor, I knew where this was going to go and I knew the time frame it was going to go in. The average life expectancy is 8 to 10 years, and all of the sudden, 10 years didn't feel like a lot of time. The further along in the journey we get, and the closer we get to what I presume to be the end of the journey, the more aware I am of time and how I spend it, especially with her. What's important now is that we make the most of what we have—each other, our children, our family and friends, and our faith—and that we make every day the best it can be."

STEPPING BACKWARD

The authors of *The 36-Hour Day* wrote that "dementia does not suddenly end a person's capacity to experience love."[1] Because people with AD do retain the capacity to experience love, incorporating the love languages into their care at every stage of the disease can help make their every day "the best day." This is not always easy, especially when the care partner is not having a "best day" of their own. The hard realities of care partnering require one to repeatedly choose to love. It is a choice that becomes more difficult and, of necessity, more intentional as each *today* fades into a yesterday. Sometimes it is helpful to pause and recall why one made this choice in the first place.

Dr. Alan Wolfelt says that when a person is grieving a death, we should not push them forward in hopes that they will quickly "get over it." Rather, he says, we should invite them to go backward to remember and honor the life of the person who died.[2] For similar reasons, reminiscing about who the PWD has been to you in years past may help you continually choose to love him or her in the future when the road may be rougher than it is right now. How did you meet him or her? What was it about him or her that you most enjoyed? Celebrate this person and what he or she has meant to your life, recalling their history, their accomplishments, and their unique personality. If you are so inclined, put these thoughts in writing so that you can reread them on "not best days" in the future. This is an important exercise because *who the person has been* is fading; who he or she will now become will be defined by the disease.

Dr. Julie Williams said that as dementia alters the personality, behaviors, and attributes of a loved one, families "have to jump through some emotional hoops as they adjust to expressing love to a *new person*—one who won't be able to reciprocate that love as they once did." Ed agrees, noting that the stronger a marriage or a family has been prior to the disease, the more positive memories there are to draw upon when love becomes a conscious daily choice. Dementia complicates every relational problem, so families and marriages that were already struggling before the disease struck may have more difficulty coping. Because the loved one is not going to be the same person they have known in the past, Dr. Williams suggests that family members prepare themselves for the probability that they "are going to feel differently" about him or her.

People early in their dementia journey can often sense that their spouses "feel differently." Timothy displayed some wry humor when he rhetorically asked his wife, "You didn't sign up for this, did you?" Danielle told her husband, "I know it's hard on you. I'm sorry." Newly diagnosed people are often also sensitive to changes in the way their spouses treat them on account of the disease. A group of married people diagnosed with early dementia shared with us their feelings about how the disease had changed their relationship with their spouse:

- Jimmy: worried about his wife's health and wonders, "Can she care for me in the future?"

- Keisha: feels that her condition "is not that bad," and is offended when her husband says he is "her caregiver."*
- Kate: sad about what her husband has to give up because of her illness, and feeling guilty about the way her life is limiting his.
- Carlos: hurt by his wife's condescending attitude.
- Geoff: "waiting to see what they will take away from me next."
- Josephine: upset that she is not seen as someone who can do things.

The consensus of the group was that their spouses were frustrated with them, and they were genuinely concerned about this. The word *poignant* comes to mind once again: those with dementia are powerless to change the course of their disease and unable to ease the frustration it causes the loved ones upon whom they must depend.

WHEN LOVE BECOMES A MOVING TARGET

Making every day the best day is a challenge, and not only because of the issues mentioned above and the caregiver burden described in the previous chapter. It is also a challenge for a reason that applies uniquely to people with AD: the love languages that are most meaningful to a person with Alzheimer's disease *change* as the disease advances.

Coco, whose father has AD, said, "Previously, when Dad and I saw each other, we always hugged and put our arms around each

---

* Keisha's comment was the impetus for our decision to use the term *care partner* instead of *caregiver* when referring to family members. *Care partner* is less hierarchical, and allows a person in the early stages of the disease to feel emotionally equal to the family member providing care.

other. Now we have to change how we show affection to a way that he can understand. Another way we used to show affection for each other was teasing back and forth. I do still try to tease with him, but now he doesn't get it, so this is not the way to do it anymore. I have to figure out how I can show my love to him in a different way now."

A change in love language was also evident in the marriage of Malik and Aisha, mentioned in chapter 2. Their marriage began to unravel when Aisha was diagnosed with mild cognitive impairment (MCI). By the time they came to see Ed, he said, "They had stopped holding hands. They had stopped cuddling. They had not been physically intimate for years." During this period of physical estrangement, Aisha's love language changed.

As is usually the case, when Malik and Aisha got married, they had different love languages. In the early years of their marriage, *Physical Touch* had been very important to Malik but not important at all to Aisha, whose love language was *Acts of Service*. Prior to Aisha's diagnosis, Malik had naturally expressed his love for her by holding hands with her, giving her hugs, and through lovemaking. When Aisha was diagnosed with MCI, Malik began to withdraw from her. As time went on, ironically, Aisha and Malik literally switched places in terms of their need for physical affection. As Aisha's disease progressed, she became distraught about the absence of physical affection in her marriage. She now needed to experience Malik's love in a way that had not been important to her in the past. In counseling, Ed taught them about the love languages and gave them homework assignments designed to rebuild their emotional connection through *Physical Touch* and *Quality Time*.

WHY LOVE LANGUAGES CHANGE

The primary love language of a cognitively healthy person does not change. If *Words of Affirmation* make a person feel loved when she is 20, they will still make her feel loved when she is 90. When AD enters the picture, however, a person's ability to perceive love becomes something of a moving target. The reason is that a particular love language can only be meaningful to a person if the brain region where it resonates has not been damaged or destroyed by the disease. As the brain deteriorates, a love language that used to be relatively unimportant to a person can become more important with the progression of the disease, as in Aisha's case. In other words, a person's perception of being loved can change as the brain itself changes.

The adult brain has about 100 billion neurons. In a healthy brain, neurons can live 100 years or longer. In a brain affected by AD, neurons become inflamed and progressively die. With the exception of a few brain regions, these dead cells are not replaced, resulting over time in many kinds of cognitive problems. Every aspect of a person's life and relationships with others is eventually impacted, including the ability to give and receive love via the five love languages.

LOVE AND THE LOBES

The first neurons to be affected by AD are in the temporal lobes of the brain in the hippocampus. The hippocampus is a seahorse-shaped structure that is essential for memory; (the name *hippocampus* comes from the Greek words, *hippos* meaning "horse" and *kampos,* meaning "sea monster"). Short-term memory loss, the hallmark symptom of Alzheimer's, is due to the loss of hippocampal neurons. From the temporal lobes, AD slowly progresses, eventually invading the frontal and parietal lobes as well. The occipital lobes, which control vision, are not usually directly impacted by AD. Not everyone experiences cognitive declines in the exact same way or at the same rate. Other types of dementia have different symptoms and may progress more quickly or slowly than AD.

While each lobe of the brain "specializes" in different things, as our friend and colleague, neuroscientist Dr. Christina Hugenschmidt, noted, "No one brain area ever works in isolation. Each area is always networking with other brain areas, so one theory is that Alzheimer's disease may spread in a network fashion."

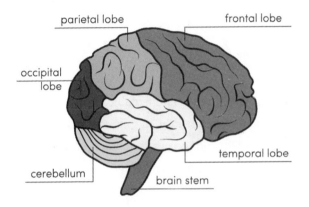

A brief glance at each lobe's key functions makes it easy to see why the love languages are impacted by Alzheimer's disease.[3,4,5,6] (For more detailed information, see "Lobes of the Brain" in Appendix B.)

Frontal Lobes: The Management Center

The frontal lobes govern executive function (the ability to pay attention, concentrate, stay on task, plan, problem solve, and multitask). These lobes are also involved in verbal expression, physical movement, and the ability to govern behavior, including inhibiting socially inappropriate words and actions. They house the mirror neurons, which enable us to empathize with others and understand their point of view.

Temporal Lobes: The Memory and Emotion Center

The temporal lobes each house a hippocampus and an amygdala. The hippocampi help form and store new memories, thus enabling us to learn. They are also important in the retrieval of long-term memories. The amygdalae govern emotion, including emotional integration, emotional learning, and emotional memory, the emotional components of stored memories. They also help us with facial recognition.

Parietal Lobes: The Internal "GPS"

The parietal lobes interpret information from our five senses and assist in the recognition of familiar objects and faces. These lobes enable us to orient ourselves in three-dimensional space, including telling right from left. Along with the temporal lobes, the parietal lobes enable mathematical skills and language comprehension.

Damaged Lobes and the Love Languages

As AD inflicts damage to the frontal, temporal, and parietal lobes, it increasingly impacts the ability to express all five love languages. Frontal lobe damage in particular can actually make a person behave in *unloving* ways. Frontal lobe damage impairs:

- Empathy, the ability to perceive and care about others' needs and feelings
- Planning and initiative, necessary for giving gifts or doing acts of service

- Expressive language, affecting one's ability to speak words of affirmation
- Motivation to express love
- Impulse control—making one prone to argue, swear, or do socially inappropriate things (called "disinhibition")
- Insight, the ability to understand that certain behaviors and comments are inappropriate, embarrassing, or hurtful to others

The expression of the love languages is also impacted by damage to the temporal and parietal lobes. Temporal lobe damage impairs many functions, including memory, the understanding of speech, recognition of faces, objects, and places, and expression of emotion.

Functions impaired by parietal lobe damage include sense of touch, spatial awareness (the "internal GPS"), recognizing or naming what is seen, and understanding what others say.

As temporal and parietal lobe damage become severe, a PWD finds it increasingly difficult to engage in quality time, receive words of affirmation, recognize family members and friends who are familiar to them, or comfortably and meaningfully experience physical touch. By the later stages of AD, when brain damage is widespread, the ability to *express* love to others is mostly lost and the ability to *receive* love via the five languages becomes "a moving target."

COMMUNICATING LOVE TO PEOPLE WITH AD

We love this quote from *The 36-Hour Day* because it expresses the key message of our book so well: "Fortunately, love is not dependent upon intellectual abilities. Focus on the ways you and others still share expressions of affection with the person who has dementia."[8] We agree, believing that at every point in the journey the focus should not be on what the person with AD has *lost*, but on what he or she still *has left*. Then the mission becomes: *given the cognition that remains, how can one best communicate love to this person?* It is so important to remember that just because individuals can no longer express love to others, it does not mean that they are unable to emotionally experience the love that others express to them.

An understanding of which of an individual's abilities have been lost helps us appropriately focus on the abilities that remain. We have looked at declining cognition in terms of brain lobe function. Let's look at it again now in the framework of the AD stages.

THE STAGES OF COGNITIVE DECLINE

Throughout the disease, amyloid plaques and tau tangles accumulate in the brain, neurons die, and the brain shrinks, leaving a person increasingly impaired. Changes occur as the disease progresses from mild to moderate to severe AD.

Mild Alzheimer's disease

In mild (early-stage) AD, though neuron death is ongoing, people still retain most functions. Early-stage AD usually lasts 2 to 4 years and is most characterized by progressive short-term memory loss. Spontaneity decreases due to apathy, and interest in spending time with family and friends may decline. Mild AD is also characterized by personality changes, impaired judgment, poor decision-making, and increasing difficulty performing tasks that require multiple steps, such as cooking or managing money. Executive function becomes impaired. Executive function is required to accomplish the relatively complex "instrumental activities of daily living" (IADLs), which are:

- Using the telephone
- Driving
- Shopping
- Preparing meals
- Doing housework and laundry
- Taking medicine
- Managing money

In very early AD, people are able to accomplish these tasks without help. As time goes on, they can still do them with some assistance. Eventually, cognition declines so much that a person is unable to do these tasks at all. When an individual is unable to perform the IADLs, they have transitioned to the middle stage of the disease and can no longer live independently.

Preclinical AD

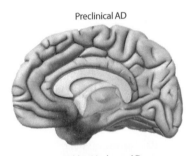

Mild to Moderate AD

Moderate (middle-stage) AD

In middle-stage AD, care partnering transitions to the more stressful *caregiving* role. As more of the brain is affected, behavioral problems and language difficulties increase and become noticeable to others. Memory loss continues, the attention span becomes shorter, and the ability to think logically wanes. Repeating, wandering,

Severe AD

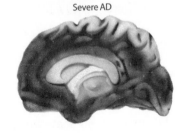

Image courtesy of the National Institute on Aging/National Institutes of Health.

delusions, disinhibition, and sundowning often occur in this longest phase of the disease, which can last 2 to 10 years.

Throughout moderate AD, people have increasing difficulty caring for and moving their own bodies. Eventually, they become unable to perform the basic "activities of daily living" (ADLs), which are less complex than the IADLs lost in early-stage AD. ADLs are the basic self-care activities that allow a person to get going in the morning, move about during the day, and prepare for bed in the evening. The ADLs are generally considered to be:

- Bathing or showering
- Dressing
- Eating
- Brushing teeth
- Toileting (bladder/bowel control and hygiene)
- Transferring (walking to sitting; sitting to lying down)

Research suggests that providing positive emotional experiences for those in this middle stage can help relieve distress and diminish behavior problems. In addition, it is comforting to know that the loss of insight into what is happening to them spares people with dementia some of the emotional anguish they might otherwise experience over their losses.

Severe (late-stage) AD

When AD has robbed a person of the ability to perform the ADLs, the disease has transitioned to severe AD, the final phase. In this stage, people lose the ability to respond to their environment. They become unable to carry on a conversation, although they may still say some words and phrases that may not be understandable. Swallowing becomes difficult and can lead to aspiration pneumonia, a type of infection that can occur if food or liquid is breathed into the lungs. They become unable to smile or tend to their own bodily needs. The ability to walk, or even sit upright in a chair, is lost, making them totally dependent upon others. This phase of the disease typically lasts from one to three years.

When people reach the final stage of AD, since they do not (cannot) respond, it seems reasonable to conclude that it is pointless to continue reaching out to them with the love languages. We understand this view, but we don't subscribe to it. One reason we don't is because of reports from people who have emerged from an unconscious state or from a coma, other conditions that keep people from responding. Consider these article excerpts:

From *Nursing Times*:

> "Lawrence (1995) found that unconscious patients could hear and respond emotionally to verbal communication. One patient, when being neurologically assessed, understood the nurse's request to squeeze her hand but was unable to move. Another stated: 'I could think and I could hear, but I could not move and I could not talk or open my eyes.'"[9]

From the UK publication *The Telegraph*:

> Geoffrey Lean wrote, "Locked in a coma after an operation went wrong, I heard medical staff discussing my case, without being able to join in. I listened to my wife talking to me, but was unable to respond . . . I could also feel my dear wife's hand in mine, our fingers entwined. I knew it was her—though I didn't really understand what she was doing there—and she brought immense reassurance."[10]

Alzheimer's expert Joanne Koenig Coste has written, "Although many losses occur with this disease, assume that the patient can still register feelings that matter."[11] It is uncommon even for a person with late-stage AD to reach a point where they are emotionally unresponsive. We believe that expressions of love continue to resonate at some deep emotional level as long as a person is alive.

SPEAKING THE LOVE LANGUAGES THROUGHOUT THE ALZHEIMER'S JOURNEY: WHY IT MATTERS

In a University of Iowa research study[12], two groups of people watched a 20-minute series of short film clips. One group had AD; the other group was cognitively normal. The first film clips made everyone sad and tearful. The second group of clips made them laugh and feel happy. After the movies ended, the participants were given a test to see what they recalled about what they had just seen. As expected, the group with AD remembered less than the other group. One person with AD didn't even remember watching the clips. But 30 minutes later, everyone in the AD group still felt sad or happy. Most significantly, the people who remembered least about the movies felt the strongest emotions.

The lead researcher told the university publication *IowaNow*, "This confirms that the emotional life of an Alzheimer's patient is alive and well."

The researchers published their findings in the journal *Cognitive and Behavioral Neurology*. They stated, "The fact that these patients' feelings can persist, even in the absence of memory, highlights the need to avoid causing negative feelings and to try to induce positive feelings with frequent visits and social interactions, exercise, music, dance, jokes, and serving patients their favorite foods. Thus, our findings should empower caregivers by showing them that their actions toward patients really do matter and can significantly influence a patient's quality of life and subjective well-being."[13]

The *IowaNow* writer saw in this study "an inescapable message: caregivers have a profound influence—good or bad—on the emotional state of individuals with Alzheimer's disease." We agree and feel that this study underscores the immense value of surrounding AD patients with positive, enjoyable, mega-doses of love, expressed in as many ways as possible.

In his foreword to *The 36-Hour Day*, Dr. Paul R. McHugh wrote that dementia, "like many other aspects of life, may follow a better or worse path depending on contexts and circumstances forged by the mediations of family and friends."[14] Whether you are a care partner, a family member, or a friend, the impact of your intentional expressions of love to a PWD cannot be overstated. Your loving gestures can infuse joy into this difficult and lonely journey.

WHEN LOVE BECOMES A ONE-WAY STREET

All love relationships are sustained by memories. "Memory is the biggest situational component of love," Ed explained. The "feeling" of love comes from the memories that we have attached to it, and this pairing occurs via the hippocampus-amygdala connection in the temporal lobe. As one partner's memory fades, the entire history of the relationship will eventually exist only in the healthy person's memory, and only he or she will be able to call forth these memories to power the relationship going forward. All people with AD not only lose the ability to create new memories with their loved one, but they also lose the memories that built the relationship in the first place. When this happens, the unaffected person is tasked with sustaining the couple's love for the remainder of the journey.

In *The 5 Love Languages*®, Gary's description of genuine love is consistently tethered to the word *choice:* love "is the *choice* to expend energy in an effort to benefit the other person;" love "grows out of reason and *choice,*" "love is always a *choice.*"[15] Choosing to love a person with AD is an extraordinarily unselfish choice. It is a choice to love someone who is—or will become—incapable of reciprocating your love, someone who cannot love you back.

Ed said, "In a relationship, you want it to be 50-50. When Rebecca's diagnosis came, I knew it was never going to be 50-50 again. Now it's like 99-1. I've been very intentional about us remaining close, even though this disease gets more and more in the way. I don't feel like my emotional love tank is full, but I know that we have maintained the best relationship possible, given the circumstances."

"When expressing love to someone with moderate or late-stage Alzheimer's disease," Ed said, "you must make the choice to love without having the expectation of being loved in return. There may not be a thank you, hug, or kiss acknowledging your loving act. Your loved one may sometimes even reject your attempt to show love to them."

You may have to remind yourself daily that your loved one is capable of receiving love.

Dr. Williams encourages people to remember that "just because you don't see a light in your loved one's eyes when you massage their feet or hold their hand, it doesn't mean this isn't connecting. It doesn't mean they don't love you." Ed agrees, acknowledging the immense difficulty of one-way love. He said, "You may have to remind yourself daily that your loved one is capable of receiving love." It's also important to celebrate any small extent to which the loved one expresses love back to you. "Your threshold for receiving love has to be dialed way down," he said.

Troy said, "One night Danielle kissed me on my shoulder. You may not get another word, another look, or anything, but at that moment, I got confirmation that she still loves me. Those are the times that get me through." Sarah's husband still sometimes says, "I love you." She said that even though "he doesn't remember our wedding," those three words "mean a lot to me now, probably more than they did before."

COMMUNICATING LOVE AS MEMORY AND COGNITION FADE

The five love languages can be used to enhance any relationship, including one with a person whose cognition is declining and whose memory is failing. Powered with kindness and creativity, the love languages can also enhance quality of life for people with AD. Dr. Hugenschmidt said it is important to remember that even if the primary love language of a PWD remains the same, "the method in which they like to receive that language might be altered."

It is also important to remember that any positive feelings generated will persist longer than the memory of the kindness that was performed. Dr. Maya Angelou once famously remarked that "people will forget what you said, people will forget what you did, but people will never forget how you made them feel."

With these two thoughts as context, let's explore some ways to use the five love languages to keep love alive throughout the Alzheimer's journey.

WORDS OF AFFIRMATION

The ability to understand language is usually preserved until late AD. For most of the journey, Dr. Williams said, "I think we have to assume that a person can receive and understand *Words of Affirmation.*"

Special Considerations

When communicating with any PWD, it is important to be respectful. Dr. Williams said, "I always address patients as though they are capable of answering all of my questions. If they stumble, I will very gently assist or ask a caregiver or family member to help with those answers." Not everyone is this sensitive to patients' feelings. Dr. Williams has observed that some people seem to think "the more they ask a question the more likely it is that the person will come up with the answer . . . What they don't realize is this is demeaning. This is an opportunity to educate families about effective communications strategies."

***

As we have seen, people with AD can experience delusional thinking. When this happens they may misinterpret verbal communication. Dr. Hugenschmidt noted, "*Words of Affirmation* is one love language that I definitely see being perceived different-ly as people progress in the disease. It seems to really change in the course of the disease because of the anxiety and suspiciousness that can go along with the brain deterioration. When this happens, *Words of Affirmation* can be perceived as being disingenuous or condescending, even threatening."

LOVE LANGUAGE *Words of Affirmation*	
Loving Considerations	**Loving *Don'ts***
EARLY AD: Focus on the feelings of the PWD rather than on facts. Saying "we" instead of "he" or "she" enhances the relationship ("We had a setback" or "We had a wonderful day"). Speak calmly, clearly, and gently. **MIDDLE TO LATE AD:** Address fear and shadowing behavior with verbal reassuarances: "I love you. You are safe, and everything is okay." Letters and cards are no longer meaningful when the PWD loses the ability to read. Even when a PWD has difficulty understanding language, they still respond to the warmth in someone's voice.	Don't drill the PWD for recall. (It won't help!) When others are present, don't speak about the PWD in the third person (he, she). Acknowledge their presence and include them in the conversation, even if they cannot verbally contribute. When the PWD is present, don't recount to others what the person can no longer do; avoid the word *can't* ("he can't do that anymore"). Don't speak to the PWD in a patronizing way as if he or she were a child ("You ate your whole meal today!"). Don't argue about their perceptions of reality. Instead of contradicting or correcting, validate their feelings and steer the conversation in another direction. Don't raise your voice or speak sharply. This can create distress.

PHYSICAL TOUCH

Physical Touch provides a wonderful way to comfort and reassure a PWD. However, as Dr. Hugenschmidt pointed out, and Ed's story in chapter 1 illustrates, "The touch that the PWD wants from you is going to change as their perception of who you are changes." Touch can be expressive or instrumental. Expressive touch consists of hugs, holding hands, stroking the hair, and other gestures of affection. Instrumental touch is task-oriented, such as occurs with the caregiving ADLs of bathing and diapering or toileting.

Special Considerations

When providing personal care, which is often first needed around the middle of the disease, it is important to do so in a way that preserves a person's dignity. The significance of this was brought home to Ed when Adele, whose mother has late-stage AD, came for a counseling visit.

"Every time I go to visit my mom in the nursing home, she hits me," Adele lamented. "Sometimes she really wallops me—hard."

Seeking to understand, Ed asked Adele some questions: what was the context for her mom's negative behavior? What seemed to trigger it?

Adele explained that she visited her mom nearly every day. The first thing she did when she arrived was change her mom's diaper. Her mother always responded by hitting Adele. This made Adele feel angry and frustrated because she was trying to be a good, nurturing daughter, just as her mother had been nurturing to her. As a result of this daily mother-daughter combat, the two spent their time together angry and interacting poorly.

Ed made two suggestions to Adele. First, delegate all diaper changing to the nursing home staff. Second, on the next visit, bring chocolate for her mom. Adele thought this seemed worth a try.

Ed recalled with satisfaction, "This new approach completely changed their relationship. It became positive. They were able to relate differently and the mother was even able to say a few words to Adele when their interaction was no longer negative." Even though Adele's mom could not walk and rarely spoke, she felt that her modesty and dignity were violated when her daughter, whose diapers she had once changed, was now changing hers. With Adele's new approach, her mother was able to receive her daughter's love through her words of affirmation, her gift of chocolate, and their quality time together.

***

When AD affects the parietal lobe, too much sensory input can be disturbing to a person with dementia. Ed said, "With Rebecca, most of the touch that occurs is at night when she goes to bed and she is snuggled under the covers. She is lying on her pillow and I think she feels safe when she's cocooned in bed. The lights are down and that's a time when she's receptive to some gentle hugging or kissing. But if I pop in after work and exclaim, 'Hi! How are you doing?' and approach her from behind and try to give her a kiss, she will be very repelled by that and will physically move away and say, 'No, no!' But if I sit in front of her and make sure she sees and hears me, I can gently hug her and offer a kiss, or two or three, and she will usually smile or laugh as she receives my affection."

***

In late-stage AD, people primarily experience life through their five senses. "Touch may . . . be the only way a patient with dementia may identify that they are receiving attention and recognition from others, which may improve their self-esteem and sense of well-being," according to the authors of a 2014 *Maturitas* article about the senses and dementia.[16]

LOVE LANGUAGE	
Physical Touch	
Loving Considerations	**Loving *Don'ts***
EARLY AD: Physical closeness tells the PWD at an emotional level, "you are not alone." Be respectful of cultural preferences about physical touch, eye contact, and personal space. **MIDDLE TO LATE AD:** Receiving many hugs at a family gathering may be too stimulating, causing the PWD to withdraw or become agitated (why one-on-one visits may work better than group visits). Combining touch with other stimulation, such as music, may also create sensory overload. At the end of life, tender touch, such as stroking the loved one's cheek, conveys love.	To preserve the dignity and modesty of the PWD, if possible don't involve family members in toileting or diapering and bathing. Instead, have same-sex paid or volunteer caregivers do this very personal caregiving. Don't forget to assess for pain. If a PWD is experiencing pain that they cannot describe, such as back pain or a headache, their response to another's touch may change.

QUALITY MOMENTS (QUALITY TIME)

In middle- to late-stage AD, it is helpful to think in terms of creating a *quality moment* instead of sharing *Quality Time*. The reframing is more accurate because life is increasingly experienced in *moments* that endure only briefly, then evaporate like a mist. There is no recollection of the past and no anticipation of the future; there is only the present moment. In the currency of time, a quality connection can occur in a moment, while quality time takes place over a span of minutes, hours, or even days, depending on the activity or adventure. Ed said, "As a care partner, you have to adapt. The focus becomes: how do I show my love for this person realizing that we are always in the moment?"

In her book, *Creating Moments of Joy,* Jolene Brackey wrote, "We are not able to create a perfectly wonderful day for those who have dementia, but it is absolutely attainable to create perfectly wonderful moments—moments that put smiles on their faces, a twinkle in their eyes, or trigger memories. Five minutes later, they won't remember what you did or said, but the feeling you left with them will linger."[17]

Special Considerations

Quality moments can actually help prolong the life of a PWD. Ed said, "One factor that causes an accelerated journey with dementia is social isolation. When someone watches a movie with Rebecca or colors with her, that social engagement is meaningful. You can tell that she loves coloring with somebody else. Her paid caregivers color right along with her probably two or three hours a day."

***

One care partner recalled, "When my wife would see an Alzheimer's commercial on TV, she was aware enough to ask tough questions: 'What is going to happen to me?' 'Are you going to leave me?' She would ask these questions over and over. It was hard to answer, but I was honest with her. I told her, 'Yes, this is what we are dealing with, but it's going to be okay. We are going to deal with it together.' Most of the time these conversations occurred when we were in bed and about to sleep, so we would cry ourselves to sleep holding each other."

This kind of intimate quality moment is much deeper than a mere shared experience. This is soul connection. *Hesed:* I am with you.

LOVE LANGUAGE *Quality Moments (Quality Time)*	
Loving Considerations	**Loving *Don'ts***
EARLY AD: Skills learned long ago, such as dancing and piano playing, are stored deep in the brain and retained for a long time. Such skills provide opportunities for sharing quality moments. Tap into the talents of the PWD for as long as possible! **MIDDLE TO LATE AD:** Join the person in whatever they are doing, even if that means picking up sticks in the yard or coloring. Music from the person's teen or young adult years may provide special comfort and enjoyment. Agitation or restlessness in the evening (sundowning) may prevent you from enjoying one another's company, for example, watching TV together. Staying with the PWD during sundowning lets them know they are not alone in their suffering.	Don't avoid answering hard questions from the PWD. Though the truth is sad, it can lead to a deeper emotional connection. Be patient if you must answer the same questions over and over. To the PWD, the question is new each time.

RECEIVING GIFTS

Dr. Hugenschmidt pointed out, "The gifts a person wants, or what constitutes a gift to them, is going to change as their function changes."

Special Considerations

In *The 5 Love Languages®*, Gary wrote, "Physical presence in the time of crisis is the most powerful gift you can give if your spouse's primary love language is *Receiving Gifts.*"[18] The diagnosis of Alzheimer's disease is certainly a crisis for any individual. For a newly diagnosed person, regardless of their love language, there is no more precious intangible gift than a spouse's assurance that they intend to keep the marriage vow "in sickness and in health."

***

Tangible gifts are most appreciated in early AD. Later, material gifts don't mean as much. Treats such as a piece of candy, as with Adele's mom, are better gifts late in the journey. Ed says that for Rebecca, "an ice cream cone is like the gift of all gifts. She loves that ice cream cone. She smiles; she chuckles. It's sometimes the highlight of my day watching her response to that gift." Prior to AD, he says, of all the love languages, receiving a gift of any kind was the least meaningful to Rebecca.

***

Sometimes, as in Ed's ice cream cone story, the gift giver experiences as much joy as the receiver. This was also true for Troy when he discreetly gave his wife, Danielle, a special gift, solely for her emotional benefit.

Since Troy is nowhere near retirement age, it is necessary for him to continue to work. To keep from having to place Danielle in a facility, he enrolled her in an adult daycare center. Danielle was reluctant to attend until Troy told her, "This is your job. This is where you work now." He gave two $20 bills to a care provider at the center and instructed her to "pay" Danielle at the end of the week.

On "payday," Troy recalled, "Danielle came out and said, 'This is all I get to work here! It's just not enough!'" Troy was amused but said, "Oh Honey, I am so sorry. Maybe we'll ask them to give you a bonus." The next week, he said, "I got 40 one-dollar bills and put them in an envelope. When Danielle came out, I asked her, 'Did they pay you today?' She said, 'Yeah!' and she's fanning all the dollars to me, and you know, she can't count money. I said, 'Wow! You got a lot of money today, didn't you?' She said, 'Yeah!' And then I'd take the money and give it back to the center for the next week."

LOVE LANGUAGE
Receiving Gifts

Loving Considerations	Loving *Don'ts*
EARLY AD: Appropriate gifts for people in early stage AD can be found online under the By Stage tab at http://store.best-alzheimers-products.com Relationship-enhancing gifts provide shared experiences: music CDs, DVD movies, coloring books and markers, 50–500 piece puzzles. **MIDDLE TO LATE AD:** Appropriate gifts for people in middle or late-stage AD can be found under the By Stage tab at http://store.best-alzheimers-products.com Material gifts are no longer important. Favorite foods or treats may be more appreciated. An iPod loaded with music is one of the most impactful of all gifts.	Don't expect the same appreciation for gifts as the person may have previously shown. By late AD, many people have difficulty recognizing objects that might have delighted them as gifts in years past. Don't give: * Lotions that might look like a beverage. * Full-length movies, difficult crossword puzzles, or novels.

ACTS OF KINDNESS (ACTS OF SERVICE)

Normally we think of an "act of service" as something utilitarian done to lighten the load of another, with the effort appreciated by the served person so much that they feel loved. Though care partners do countless acts of service for people with AD—administering medications, helping them dress, etc.—the PWD is not likely to appreciate the effort or perceive it as love. Dr. Williams said that for people with dementia, *Acts of Service* can be redefined "in a new way, to include preserving individuality and identity." In chapter 2, Sally's acts of service for her husband included arranging for him to accomplish tasks like "mowing" the yard and walking their dog, which make him feel useful. Dr. Williams described Sally's effort on behalf of her husband as "an act of kindness."

LOVE LANGUAGE *Acts of Kindness (Acts of Service)*	
Loving Considerations	**Loving *Don'ts***
EARLY AD: Be aware that *Acts of Service* may remind a PWD of their own inability to express love through an act of service, such as cooking a meal.	Don't discourage a PWD who wants to help. Find small tasks they can do, such as folding towels, or "washing" dishes so they feel they are making a contribution.
MIDDLE TO LATE AD: Realize that doing acts of service for a PWD will not convey the same meaning it once did. Think in terms of doing *acts of kindness* rather than acts of service.	Whenever possible, do *with* rather than *for*.

MID- TO LATE-STAGE AD:
SPEAKING ALL THE LOVE LANGUAGES

In *The 5 Love Languages® of Children,* Gary and coauthor Ross Campbell suggest that while parents should try to identify their child's primary love language, they should also deliberately speak all five love languages with their child. They say, "Yes, we believe your child perceives love best from one of the five languages, but the other four ways of showing your love will also benefit them."[19]

In the middle and late stages of AD, people become more childlike. Ed recalled, "Once when Carrie, our youngest daughter, was home, she spent an evening with Rebecca, then tucked her mom into bed. Rebecca looked up at Carrie and said, 'It was so much fun playing with the big kids today.' At this stage in her disease, Rebecca was clearly perceiving life from the point of view of a child. Because people with mid- to late-stage AD do regress to a more childlike state of mind, we suggest expressing love to them as if they were, in fact, children. Taking our cue from Drs. Chapman and Campbell, we recommend speaking all five love languages with those rendered childlike by dementia. We also think this is a prudent approach since a person's love language can change throughout the disease. When no particular love language stands out as primary, expressing love in five different ways only increases the chances of hitting the target!

Our friend Troy does an excellent job of speaking all five love languages to his wife, Danielle. Troy now lives with Danielle in a memory care unit, but he often brings her to their former residence, which he still maintains, for "Danielle Day."

Years before AD struck, Danielle and Troy heard someone named Gary Chapman speak on a topic they had never heard of before: the five love languages. They enjoyed his seminar, bought the book, and each took the quiz to determine their love languages. Most couples have different love languages but both Troy and Danielle's primary and secondary love languages were the same. *Quality Time* was primary and *Physical Touch* was secondary for both. On Danielle Day, Troy now continues to speak *Quality Time* and *Physical Touch* to Danielle and lavishes her with generous doses of the other three languages as well.

"Our Danielle Days consist of me doting on her and loving on her. I get her home and I have some stuff she likes to snack on, and I feed her and make small talk. Just about every other minute I am telling her that I love her. Then I shower her and get her cleaned up. I put lotion on her feet and hands and put a hot cloth on her face. She is so at peace when all of this is going on. She just relaxes and sits. Then I lotion her face and shave her legs. I give her a top-to-bottom massage, just loving on her. And then I'll cook her a meal. It's a time that we sit together and she'll just look at me and smile so big. You know, it's just all-day love."

If you provide care for a person who is very impaired or no longer verbal, your best clues about what makes them feel loved *right now* may be their current behaviors and preferences. This requires guesswork, but by reassessing periodically, you may be able to continually recognize the best way to express love to them in the moment. At any point in the latter half of the disease, or at any point when no particular love language emerges as primary, we offer the list in Appendix A as a creative starting point for speaking all five love languages.

5

Facilitating Love

"There is nothing more beautiful than someone
who goes out of their way to make life beautiful for others."
—MANDY HALE

IN THE NATURAL SCHEME of things, expressions of love reward both the giver and the receiver. When others express love to us in our "native tongue" (our love language), our emotional love tank begins to fill and life feels good. When we reach out to others in the same way, with expressions of love designed just for them, we feel good about what we have done, and if the other person responds with appreciation or surprise or pleasure, we feel even better because their response rewards our effort. When love is spoken in the appropriate languages, and flows freely in both directions, giving love is as rewarding as receiving it. In fact, human beings are innately wired to enjoy this reciprocal kind of love.

THE NATURAL REWARD FOR SHOWING LOVE TO OTHERS

When we see that our loving gesture has impacted another person as we had hoped, it triggers the release of the "feel-good" chemical dopamine from special neurons in the brain's reward pathway. This natural reward helps motivate us to repeat whatever we have done. The more we see that our expressions of love are meaningful to other people, the more we feel rewarded, and the more we want to keep on showing love.

"In terms of your love language," Dr. Christina Hugenschmidt told us, "it's whatever you find rewarding. For example, what makes you excited about giving a gift is seeing the person's face light up. The other person's response to the gift is the reward." (We would be remiss if we did not point out that it is the very *absence* of such responses from people with dementia that makes care partners' selfless *hesed* love so impressive.)

> In the natural scheme of things, expressions of love reward both the giver and receiver.

Until key components of the brain's reward system are impaired by AD, people remain quite capable of experiencing the satisfaction and joy that come from expressing love to others. The problem is that while they have the capacity to *enjoy* the reward that comes from reaching out to others, they are increasingly challenged in their ability to *initiate* expressions of love. They become unable to remember the sequence of tasks that leads to the reward, and are increasingly unable to perform the tasks themselves. In order to express love to another person, people with AD need the help of a *facilitator*, someone who is motivated to step in and assist.

FACILITATING FOR PEOPLE WITH DEMENTIA

The Memory Counseling Program that Ed founded includes a "Brain Fitness" group for people with dementia. Brain Fitness provides cognitive and emotional stimulation through social engagement, art, music, interactive games, and dance. Facilitators help those with dementia to engage in creative activities that enhance their quality of life. Sometimes this involves one of the love languages. Consider these examples:

In one Brain Fitness group, the activity was painting, so the facilitators brought in flowers to give the participants something to paint. Afterward, group members were told they could each give a flower to their care partner when that person arrived to pick them up. When Aaron's wife, Sandra, arrived, he enthusiastically grabbed the whole bunch of flowers and gave it to her. Sandra, of course, realized that all of the flowers were not meant for her. Dr. Hugenschmidt, the group leader, recalled, "She felt awkward about it. But we said, 'Please take them because this has made him so happy.' The other care partners were also saying, 'Take the flowers!'

"Aaron was so excited to be able to give something to his wife, and he can't do that on his own. Maybe he would have liked to have gotten flowers for Sandra many times, but he cannot drive; he cannot plan anymore; he has a hard time initiating. But when the flowers are right there and someone says, 'You can give those to Sandra,' his face lights up! I think part of what he enjoyed was that it was something he felt that he had done on his own, because it happened outside of his connection with Sandra. She didn't take him to the store to get flowers; he was with his group. He had flowers to give her when she walked into the room. That was really important to him."

Dr. Hugenschmidt continued, "When there is a non-primary care partner to facilitate, the person with AD can have that feeling of independence and experience the reward of the surprise. Otherwise, the care partner has to help them get the gift and I think that's disappointing for the care partner and for the person with dementia. It's like the situation with a single mom whose child wants to do something for his mom's birthday. How does that happen? A lot of times it's someone else in the family or a friend who recognizes that, takes the child to the store, and helps them get a gift so they can have that joy of being able to surprise the person they love."

***

The Brain Fitness leaders have noticed that several of the group's participants have trouble with expressive language. When a person is not verbally expressive, it's easy to assume that they would not respond to a facilitator's efforts. Dr. Hugenschmidt said, "Many people mistake an inability to express for an inability to receive. And that is not necessarily the case. One of our participants, Paula, has a lot of problems with expression. She used to be a poet and do poetry readings. I can only imagine how frustrating it is to be that fluent with words and then not be able to generate them. As a group, we wrote a haiku and we asked her to be the reader. We chose her because she can read and she can say the words she reads, but she just can't generate words herself. Reading the haiku to the group gave her an opportunity to be expressive without having to self-generate the words. She really seemed to like doing this."

As a pre-dementia poet, it is not hard to see why reading the haiku was rewarding for Paula. However, she could not have created this reading opportunity for herself. It had to be created for her and facilitated by the group's leadership. "If you were Paula's care partner," Dr. Hugenschmidt noted, "you might underestimate what she can do or what she can understand or engage with, because she can't verbally tell you. If her primary love language is *Words of Affirmation,* it would be a mistake to quit talking to her because she can still receive words very well."

***

The authors of *The 36-Hour Day* wrote that "*much can be done to improve the quality of life of people who have dementia and their family members*" [emphasis in original].[1] Facilitating activities that encourage self-expression is one way to improve quality of life for people with dementia. Self-expression increases self-efficacy, one's belief in his own ability to complete tasks and reach goals. Since the abilities of people with dementia are constantly declining, facilitating the things they can still do builds self-efficacy.

"One thing we have noticed in Brain Fitness," said Dr. Hugenschmidt, "is that people's skills deteriorate a lot in the realm of planning and remembering or being able to initiate. With one woman, Hannah, who is a painter, we watched these deteriorate markedly. Nevertheless, she still enjoys painting. It's just that the infrastructure that it takes for her to paint now is different. It used to be that she would buy her paints and canvases, choose what she wanted to paint, drive over to be with her friends, and paint in a group. Now you have to buy the materials for her; you have to give her a model; and sometimes you have to put the paintbrush into her hand and put the paints out for her. But when you do that, she still paints and she still enjoys it.

"I think the inability to initiate can be misinterpreted as a loss of function, when all that's really needed is just a facilitator— someone who has the time and the energy and the patience to step in and fill in the gaps, understanding that the original passion or enjoyment is still there but the person can't act on it without help," Dr. Hugenschmidt said.

FACILITATING GIVING GIFTS AND ACTS OF SERVICE

Because the executive functions of planning, taking initiative, and sequencing are lost in early AD, the love languages that most require these abilities—giving gifts and doing acts of service—are the first expressions of love to be impaired by the disease. As illustrated by the story about Aaron and the flowers, a person's ability to give gifts can be prolonged only with the help of a facilitator. The ability to do acts of service can also be prolonged with the help of a facilitator, if the focus is on the self-efficacy that is generated by doing tasks, rather than on the quality of the work. For example, Sarah said her husband always "wants to help, so on laundry day, I let him fold all the towels. They're not folded very well and he puts them in the closet any which way they will go as long as he can jam them onto the shelf."

Many people seem to retain a strong desire to continue expressing these two love languages in particular long after their capacity to do so is gone.

THE DESIRE TO CONTINUE GIVING

Dr. Hugenschmidt said, "People who are really motivated to give gifts still give gifts. It's just that the gifts are much less appropriate. Without facilitation, gift giving can sometimes cause a lot of sadness for the care partner because they see that the person still loves them and is really trying. It's just that the trying is a failure." (Care partners may find it helpful to think of any gift from a PWD as they would a gift from a young child, focusing more on the giver's intent than the gift itself.)

Though they remain motivated to give, people with dementia don't have much they can actually give. One of the only things they *can* give is the food they "own." When Rebecca Shaw was at an earlier point in her disease, she once broke off a piece of taco shell from the taco salad she was eating, handed it to Ed, and said, "This is for you." Ed immediately recognized that this was a gift.

Dr. Julie Williams said, "Many individuals who are starting to enter the disinhibition phase of their disease want to share their hospital food with the doctors or nurses or medical students. They'll say, 'This is really good banana pudding, but I'm too full. Would you like to have the rest?' or 'I've got some grapes here. Help yourself!'" This desire to continue giving may persist long into the disease. Dr. Williams said, "In the hospital, if someone has very advanced disease and is minimally verbal, she might pick up an object within reach, a utensil, an item of food, or a magazine, and hand it to a visitor. The person receiving it usually has no idea what is going on and might say, 'Why are you giving me this?' but a very perceptive person will say, 'Thank you so much. It's perfect. I will put it right here.'"

THE DESIRE TO CONTINUE SERVING

Some people whose primary pre-dementia love language was *Acts of Service* have a strong desire to continue serving others, even as their disease advances. Rebecca Shaw is one of these people. Ed said, "Rebecca grew up without a dishwasher and prefers to wash dishes by hand. Even when we had a dishwasher she often would do dishes by hand. After supper either her caregivers or I will help her get the dishes into the sink and she will 'wash the dishes.' She's not really capable of washing them in a way that makes them ready for use, so after she goes to bed we put them in the dishwasher. Rebecca has retained the desire to serve her family with the one last act of service that she can still do, which is dishwashing."

Rebecca's desire to wash dishes remains in play even when she is not at home. One evening Ed, Rebecca, and four members of "The A Team" (her paid caregivers) went to a restaurant for supper. After the meal, Rebecca grabbed her empty plate and arose from the table, heading for the restaurant kitchen, presumably to help with the dishes! Ed and the caregivers had to follow and convince her to abandon her mission.

In the early years of their marriage, Sarah recalled, "Bob always wanted to help me." Now, although he can no longer help, he still wants to pitch in. Sarah said, "When I'm in the kitchen making dinner, he says, 'Here I am sitting doing nothing and you're doing all the work. I should be helping you.' He will tell me this probably three or four times while I am preparing dinner. I think that is his way of showing love."

Sarah and Bob's daughter, Coco, also recognizes her dad's desire to continue showing love through *Acts of Service,* despite his inability to actually do so. However, facilitating an act of service for her dad is not always convenient. Coco explained, "Dad wanted to help with the dishes last night. Sometimes I feel that he's like a kid, like when your kids are toddlers and they are trying to help you do things and it's easier to say, 'Just let me do it.' That's what I did last night. He just stood there. If I had handed him the dish and let him put it in the dishwasher it would have been fine." In retrospect, she said, "I feel that in order to keep his emotional tank full, as hard as it is, I should let him help, because that's what keeps him happy."

FACILITATING QUALITY TIME, TOUCH, AND WORDS

As the Brain Fitness examples of painting and reading haiku show, facilitating for those with dementia can enable them to continue doing something they enjoy after they have lost the ability to do it on their own. Similarly, a person with dementia can continue experiencing and expressing the love languages of *Quality Time*, *Physical Touch*, and *Words of Affirmation* for a longer time if a facilitator is willing to participate along with them. Touch speaks simultaneously to the person doing the touching and the person being touched. By picking up a person's hand as you talk, or putting your arm around them in the movies or in church, you are not only speaking the love language, but also facilitating its passive expression, as both people are touching. This is also true of *Quality Time* because both the facilitator and the person with dementia are experiencing it together, one speaking the love language actively and the other passively.

Dr. Hugenschmidt said, "Often *Quality Time* means a certain activity for people, like going to the movies or riding bikes, but if you can be flexible about how the time is spent, the window for experiencing *Quality Time* will remain open a little longer." For both small children and people with AD, prolonging *Quality Time* often means that the care partner must be willing to repeat the same activity many, many times. "With two-year-olds," Dr. Hugenschmidt said, "you're going to read that favorite book to them over and over. It may not be personally rewarding for you to read *Marvin K. Mooney, Will You Please Go Now?* for the hundredth time, but that's your quality time." Reading a book also facilitates physical closeness between parent and child, and allows them to share a *Words* experience. Ed's quality time with Rebecca mirrors this parent-child experience, except that the *Words* experience is song lyrics and movie dialogue.

He said, "Rebecca is fairly touch averse, but when we watch a DVD she will let me touch her. Sometimes I'll lock my arm in hers. Once in a while she will even let me hold her hand, but we will always be thigh to thigh, if you will, sitting on the couch. *The Sound of Music* is her favorite musical. I think I have seen it literally hundreds of times. These movie nights allow love to be expressed through *Physical Touch* and *Quality Time*, doing something together that we both enjoy."

FACILITATING LOVE THROUGH MUSIC

Henry Wadsworth Longfellow said, "Music is the universal language of mankind." Music is not one of the five love languages, but with its own system of notation, music easily meets the dictionary definition of a *language*: "the system of words or signs that people use to express thoughts and feelings to each other."[2] As Mr. Longfellow opined, music is the one language that uniquely resonates with all of humanity.

Through the centuries and across cultures, music has provided entertainment, lulled babies to sleep, enhanced celebrations, and expressed the praises of worshipers. Medically, it has long been known that music has a positive impact on blood pressure, cortisol, dopamine, melatonin, and oxygen levels, and helps alleviate depression and anxiety. Now, as the Alzheimer's epidemic begins its crescendo, the healing power of music is gaining new attention. Many research studies have highlighted the therapeutic effects of music on Alzheimer's patients, reducing aggression, anxiety, and agitation while improving mood and behavior.[3,4,5,6,7] Newer research strongly suggests that music can also improve cognition. Linda Maguire, an opera singer with master's degrees in both neuroscience and health science/gerontology, conducted a study that showed "remarkable improvements in cognition" after people with AD sang a regimen of her handpicked songs for four months. Ms. Maguire told *Epoch Times,* "Music gives Alzheimer's patients a sense of power and ownership. They can't follow life. They can't follow conversations. They don't remember people . . . But because the part of the brain that internalizes music and marks rhythm particularly is very healthy in Alzheimer's patients they can follow music, and remember it, and that makes them feel in control."[8]

Singing activates both sides of the brain. Enjoying music in a group setting engages the visual areas of the brain as well. Thus, music stimulates many cognitive processes at once, in fact, more than any other known stimulus, according to world-renowned neurologist Dr. Oliver Sacks. Sometimes introducing music to a person with AD via an iPod and headphones elicits an astonishing response. Thousands of people have marveled at a video of a man named Henry, a resident of a care facility for ten years, who was uncommunicative until music made him "come alive." You can watch the video at YouTube.com by searching for "Alive Inside Henry's Story." When asked, "What does music do to you?", Henry responds, "It gives me the feeling of love." The clip of Henry is an excerpt from *Alive Inside*, a moving documentary that won the Audience Award at the 2014 Sundance Film Festival.

Alzheimer's products blogger Dan Schmid wrote, "Sometimes music brings on a change that is so amazing that we feel compelled to recommend to you, as a care provider, keep music in your repertoire." [9] Because the ability to appreciate music endures so long, and the response can be so profound, we suggest pairing music with the love languages throughout the Alzheimer's journey to enhance one's personal connection with a PWD:

Gifts

An iPod loaded with music from the person's younger years may be one of the best gifts that can be given to a person with AD. "Reminiscence" music (from one's childhood, teen years, and early adulthood) is most likely to resonate deeply. In early- to mid-AD, choose music the person enjoyed as a young adult (ages 18–25). As the person regresses to a more childlike state, load the iPod with sing-along songs and other music for children. If English is not the person's first language, try to find music in the language he or she spoke as a child. Observe the person's response to the music. If a certain song stimulates joy, keep it; if it causes sadness or agitation, delete it.

Words of Affirmation (Lyrics)

It is surprising but true that people with moderate or severe AD can often learn new song lyrics or accurately sing those learned long ago. This ability usually remains until very late in the disease because musical memory is not significantly impacted by AD. An inspiring example is country singer Glen Campbell, who completed a 15-month, 151-show concert tour as his AD progressed. This final concert tour of his career was chronicled in the 2011 CNN Films documentary, "I'll Be Me."

Physical Touch

Music invites toe tapping, clapping, and touch. As long as people are able to walk, they can sway to music holding onto someone else, or even dance with them. If music evokes memories from a couple's courting days, dancing together may inspire some hugs, handholding, and kisses too. The enjoyment of music plus touch can facilitate relational intimacy.

Quality Time

Music that encourages playful socialization can create quality time or at least quality moments. Music therapist Loretta Quinn recommends songs such as 'The Hokey Pokey' because such music "guides them to look, laugh and talk with other people around them."[10] Be sensitive to the possibility of overstimulation, taking care to eliminate noisy competition, such as from a TV or radio.

Acts of Service

Whenever love is expressed by pairing music with one of the other love languages, *Acts of Service* is always also involved because introducing music to a PWD requires at least one other person's participation.

MUSIC AND CARE PARTNERING

In *This Is Your Brain on Joy*, Dr. Earl Henslin wrote, "Lyrics coupled with the sounds of music tend to bypass the thinking part of the brain and go straight to the mood center."[11] This is as true for care partners as it is for people with AD. Music can provide stress relief for care partners. Besides this calming and joy-producing personal benefit, music can also play a role in helping care partners manage the behavior and daily care of a person with AD. Connie Tomaino, founder of the Institute for Music and Neurologic Function, told an *AARP* interviewer that when someone is in the early stages of Alzheimer's, care partners should begin associating specific songs with family members or important ideas. Later in the disease, she says, playing or singing those songs may trigger that association.[12]

The author of the *AARP* article, Mary Ellen Geist, wrote that when she and her mother were caring for her father, who had AD, "we used music in every aspect of caregiving. I sang or played Frank Sinatra's 'In the Wee Small Hours of the Morning' to wake him up. Instead of being lost and confused in the mornings, as often happens for people with Alzheimer's, the song made him realize where he was and who my mother and I were . . . Jazz classics like George Gershwin's 'Summertime' and Cole Porter's 'Night and Day' were great for showering, brushing teeth and getting dressed. I used the songs to distract him during these tasks. In the afternoons, when what's called 'sundowning' sometimes occurs and Alzheimer's patients get anxious or angry, Diana Krall's version of 'I Get Along Without You Very Well' would calm him down."[12]

FACILITATING LOVE THROUGH COUNSELING

Research suggests that when a dementia patient and their care partner are counseled together, outcomes are better for both people. According to Mary Mittelman, a research professor at NYU School of Medicine, when spouses are treated as equals by a counselor, the communication between them improves because the healthy spouse no longer discounts the one with AD, and the spouse with AD no longer shuts down emotionally.[13] This is part of the rationale for offering counseling to those dealing with dementia.

When Ed's wife was diagnosed with AD, his quest for emotional support opened his eyes to the paucity of resources available to most families. In response, he sought additional training in mental health counseling, then founded a counseling program that meets four critical client needs: "talk therapy" (psychotherapy), education (psychoeducation), relationship building, and problem solving. *Psychotherapy* means speaking one-on-one with a counselor or with others in a support group. This "talk therapy" helps people deal with the emotions, worries, and behaviors that arise during the Alzheimer's journey. *Psychoeducation* means educating people about dementia and empowering them to deal with their situation in the best possible way. An analysis of 78 interventions for care partners of older adults found that these two things—psy-

> When we feel disconnected from those we love, we experience distress, panic, and grief, and naturally seek reconnection.

choeducation and psychotherapy—were most consistently effective across all of the short-term outcomes that were measured.[14]

ATTACHMENT AND THE FIVE LOVE LANGUAGES

Many of the relationship challenges of AD occur because the disease weakens the attachment bonds between loved ones. These deep natural relationship bonds begin at birth and continue throughout life. When we feel disconnected from those we love, we experience distress, panic, and grief, and naturally seek reconnection. As Alzheimer's advances, and the attachments between loved ones weaken, the PWD often reacts with fear, agitation, or even aggression. Care partners may respond to them with anger, frustration, or by isolating. This creates division—exactly the opposite of what their loved one with dementia needs.

"Understanding attachment is fundamental to effectively counseling those on the dementia journey," said Ed. (For more information, see "Attachment" in Appendix B.)

RELATIONSHIP COUNSELING AND
THE FIVE LOVE LANGUAGES

Relationship issues resulting in discord between marriage partners, parents and their adult children, or among siblings or other family members, are among the most common challenges seen in the Memory Counseling Program. To facilitate relationship building, Ed often seeks to discover or introduce the love languages of those he counsels.

"The five love languages are problem-solving tools for helping loved ones maintain, strengthen, or even reestablish as much connection as possible," he said, "despite the fact that this disease is, using the tapestry metaphor, relentlessly unraveling the attachments that are vital to one's identity as a parent, sibling, spouse, adult child, or friend. They help build relational intimacy by facilitating both the giving and the receiving of emotional love."

Ed begins the counseling process by listening to the PWD and their care partner(s) describe how the disease has impacted their relationships: individually, as a couple, and for their family. This may take several sessions. Once the relational challenges are identified, it is important for clients to gain at least a basic understanding of the five love languages in order to utilize them as tools for relationship growth and development. If the PWD is beyond mild cognitive impairment and into early-stage Alzheimer's, retaining information about the love languages may be challenging because of short-term memory loss. In this case, Ed takes a love language inventory informally. In conversation, he attempts to discover the clients' primary love languages: before dementia, how did the PWD express love to others? What did he or she complain about most, revealing unmet desires? What requests did he or she most often make of others? The story of Frank and Shirley illustrates how Ed has utilized this process with struggling couples.

Frank was diagnosed with early-stage AD several years before he and Shirley were seen in the counseling program. By the time they sought counsel they had "grown miles apart." Shirley took the love languages quiz and identified *Quality Time* as her primary love language. With her help, Frank also took the quiz and also identified *Quality Time* as his primary love language. Frank, an introvert who loved to read, was unaware that Shirley, an extrovert, was feeling increasingly isolated, alone, and unloved as he spent more and more time each day reading and less time with her.

As Ed often does when counseling couples, he asked Shirley and Frank to face one another while Shirley shared her feelings. Frank admitted he had no idea Shirley had been feeling this way, and he apologized with tears in his eyes. With little short-term memory, Frank simply couldn't remember or keep track of how much (or little) time he and Shirley spent together in a day. With Ed's gentle facilitation, as Shirley learned to sit beside Frank while he read, and Frank readily agreed to join Shirley on errands or activities in their retirement community, they both began to feel more loved by the other.

Unlike Frank and Shirley's situation, when the PWD's primary love language has been changed by the disease, a more challenging situation results.

FACILITATING LOVE WHEN
LOVE LANGUAGES HAVE CHANGED

When the natural love language of the PWD has changed due to disease progression, Ed guides the care partner to express love using whatever love languages are still operational for the person with dementia. This response to the "moving target" of chang-ing love languages can be illustrated using ballroom dancing as a metaphor. The couple is dancing, with the PWD taking the lead and the healthy partner adapting their steps as the music—the disease—repeatedly requires them to change the routine, or for our purposes, change the love language. This "love them where they're at" approach is how Ed worked with Malik, whose wife, Aisha, experienced a love language change (chapter 4). It is always the care partner, not the person with the disease, who must do all the changing and adapting—modifying the metaphorical "dance steps" of the love relationship.

CONFRONTING THE DELUSION OF UNFAITHFULNESS

Ed sometimes uses the love languages to address relationship problems directly caused by Alzheimer's disease. This was how he facilitated a solution for Nick and Norma, a couple dealing with the paranoid delusion of marital unfaithfulness.

Norma, who has AD, was plagued by the delusion that her husband, Nick, was unfaithful to her. Although delusions do not usually occur until middle-stage AD or later, this particular delu-sion had been unusually prominent for Norma even early in her disease. Sometimes simply being at a social gathering with other couples was enough to trigger her suspicion that Nick was un-faithful. She worried constantly that Nick would find a lover—or that maybe he already had one.

As Norma's illness progressed, Nick needed the help of a day-time caregiver. Norma became extremely distressed one day when she saw Nick and her caregiver talking, assuming, of course, that they were involved with each other. Nick was, and had always been, innocent of the unfaithfulness that Norma had imagined throughout her illness. But because delusions seem real to the person experiencing them, even though Norma and Nick had a physically intimate relationship, Norma felt unloved and insecure. No amount of reasoning or explanation from Nick could comfort her. This was a crisis issue they brought to Ed in counseling.

Although Norma's delusional thinking was generated by her dementia, her feeling that Nick did not love her was not entirely without merit, as Ed discovered.

"What I learned from meeting with Norma was that *Words of Affirmation* is number one for her and every other love language is a distant second," he said. Ed recognized that Norma's delusion of unfaithfulness was made worse by her empty emotional tank. After she and her husband would be physically intimate, Ed said, "Nick would just get out of bed and go do the next thing on his checklist without even saying anything to her," said Ed. "She would have a lot of emotional 'warm fuzzies' from their time together, but she received no verbal affirmation from Nick during or after lovemaking. She concluded that he really didn't love her because he just walked away." Ed saw that "this really left her with what was, in a sense, an open emotional wound, the feeling that she and Nick were unattached."

"The way to heal that wound," said Ed, "was helping Nick understand that Norma needed to *hear* that he loved her, and she needed to hear this in the context of their lovemaking. He was completely oblivious to the fact that she felt this way and it was clear that he did not understand her love language." Ed said, "Counseling made Nick aware of what a love language is, first of all, and then what Norma's primary love language was, and how he could 'speak it' in their relationship."

"It really did help them," said Ed. "This became a non-issue for them because Nick became very intentional about the way he expressed love to Norma, understanding that she needed cuddling *with the words, "I love you,"* during and after lovemaking. He also began to affirm her verbally in between the times when they made love."

FACILITATING UNITY

Because many care partners do not have access to dementia-specific counseling, we would like to share a strategy for dealing with delusional thinking, agitation, or other negative behaviors. This strategy, which Ed calls *Acknowledge, Affirm, Redirect,* is a simple, three-step approach that gives care partners a way to diffuse potentially volatile issues, such as Norma's delusion of infidelity. Here's how it works:

In a hypothetical scenario similar to the one above, Dan, the AD patient, accuses his wife, Marian, of infidelity. Marian, feeling hurt, lashes out at Dan, saying, "How could you ever say that I would cheat on you? It offends me to my core! I have been faithful to you for 50 years and for you to even think that I would cheat on you . . . I can't even be in the same room as you!" But if Marian, recognizing that *this truly is the disease speaking,* takes a moment to compose herself, she could instead:

Acknowledge: "Dan, I hear you saying that you are worried that I am seeing somebody else."

Affirm: "Well, let me reassure you, we've been married 50 years; I've been faithful to you for 50 years, and there is nothing that is going to change that."

Redirect: "So let's go sit on the couch together and turn on the TV and have a little popcorn."

ALTERNATE RESPONSES

Acknowledge, Affirm, Redirect becomes even more effective when it incorporates the love languages in the "affirm" and "redirect" portions of this framework. For example, if Marian knows that Dan is most responsive to the love language of *Gifts*, she might hold out her hand, displaying her wedding ring, and say, "Look at my wedding ring, Dan. You gave this to me. It is a precious gift. I could never cheat on you."

If Dan responds best to *Physical Touch*, Marian might take his hand or stroke his cheek or even embrace him while she is speaking. If Dan's love language is *Words of Affirmation*, Marian might reassure Dan as in the examples above, adding comments such as, "I took a vow with you and when we said 'till death do us part,' I meant it. I would never want to be with anyone but you." If Dan responds best to *Quality Time*, Marian's redirect above is a good example. She defuses the situation with a suggestion to spend some quality time together, sitting down to watch TV and enjoy some popcorn.

Other redirects might be:

Words of Affirmation: "Let's pull out our wedding album and I will read our vows to you."

Receiving Gifts: "Why don't we use that gift card the kids gave us for our anniversary and go out to dinner?"

Physical Touch: "How about if you sit in your favorite chair while I give you a foot massage?"

Music: Begin singing a song that has been meaningful to the person with dementia, or to the marriage relationship.

FACILITATING RECONNECTION

Let's return now to the story of Malik and Aisha. After Aisha's diagnosis of MCI, household duties and cooking became more and more difficult for her, so Malik assumed most of these responsibilities. Because Aisha's primary love language was *Acts of Service*, doing these tasks had been very meaningful for her, and she missed doing them. With the emotional gulf between her and Malik widening, and the growing loss of these meaningful activities, Aisha became depressed. When the emotional pain became too great, they sought counseling.

As you may recall, as Aisha's cognition changed over time, so did her love language. Now that *Physical Touch* had become more important to Aisha than *Acts of Service*, Ed saw *Physical Touch* as the way to facilitate their reconnection.

Touch did in fact become the "emotional glue" that reconnected them to one another. As the couple completed the homework which Ed had assigned to them in a series of counseling appointments, Malik again drew close to Aisha. Using his own natural primary love language of touch, he reached out to hold her hand, snuggle with her, and put his arm around her. As Aisha regained confidence in Malik's love, her depression faded. When the couple returned for a follow-up counseling visit, Malik told Ed, "Our relationship keeps improving. We now lie close to one another when we go to bed, facing each other. We hold hands wherever we go. We have learned that we hold each other up, not just to steady the other, as we're both unsteady on our feet, but emotionally too."

Reflecting on this moment with Malik and Aisha, Ed said, "It was sweet."

FACILITATING FAMILY ISSUES

When the PWD Denies Their Disease

Some individuals will contend, with sincerity and vigor, that they don't have dementia. Michael declared, "There is nothing wrong with my brain! I don't understand why the doctors feel compelled to give me some sort of diagnosis when I occasionally forget someone's name. I thought that was normal for someone 68 years old!"

Though extremely frustrating for all concerned, one of two things usually explains a reaction like Michael's. Dementia often affects the part of the brain that gives us insight, the ability to understand a situation or condition. The lack of insight explains why some with dementia are not sad or angry about it. For others, insight is preserved, which is why many with the disease *are* depressed, anxious, and/or angry as they do realize what their brain can't do anymore. Alternatively, the person with dementia might also be in denial. Denying a painful reality is a way to bury the situation in one's unconscious mind.

With an understanding of the "why" behind Michael's statement, his wife can respond in a truthful yet loving way: "I'm sorry, Honey. It must be frustrating to be told that you have Alzheimer's when you don't see yourself as being any different than you were before. We'll get through this together." Ed counsels patients and families not to avoid saying the "D word" (dementia) or the "A word" (Alzheimer's). Saying these words teaches people that they can openly express their emotions about the disease.

Why Should I Visit if She Doesn't Remember Me?

In a family counseling session, a 28-year-old daughter whose mother has early-onset AD and is in a memory care unit (locked assisted living facility) tearfully said to her father, "Why does it matter if I visit Mom? She won't remember I was there, and besides, she doesn't even know who I am anymore."

Ed responds to this frequently asked question by first acknowledging the feelings involved. He tells families, "Just entering a long-term care facility is difficult. The sights and smells can trigger guilt about having placed our loved one there, and fears about what our own future may hold." Next, he shares the notion of *hesed*, intentional love: we visit because it is the loving thing to do. He tells family members, "Even though the person with dementia likely won't be able to remember who you are or how they know you, they are fully able to receive your love. Just by choosing to visit, you have given the gift of your time."

He offers these tips:

- Sit as close to your loved one as possible.
- Hold hands or place a gentle hand on the person's shoulder or elbow.
- Make eye contact. Human beings communicate trust and safety by looking at one another.
- Talk about old photos or family stories. Most people even with advanced dementia retain some connection to their past, so reminiscing can be affirming.

Ed reminds them, "Even if you get no response, remember that a loved one with dementia, like any other human being, needs emotional connection. Remember also that a visit is not solely for the person with dementia; it is also for the visitor. At the end of the journey, each of us who has been part of the life of a loved one with dementia wants to look back and feel we've done the best we could for them."

Facilitating the Long-Term Care Placement Decision

Art and Delia had enjoyed 40 years of marriage and raised three children. Delia, an elementary school teacher once named Teacher of the Year, began having memory problems that were apparent to her students as well as her colleagues. Delia's principal expressed concern about her ability to continue in the classroom. Both Art and Delia were shocked when Delia, age 62, was diagnosed with early-onset Alzheimer's disease. Within a year after retirement, Delia's short-term memory was gone. She couldn't speak intelligibly and got lost walking in the neighborhood. She needed help getting dressed, and had bladder accidents day and night. When Art tried to help Delia clean up and change her clothes, she became verbally abusive and physically aggressive. Having her husband put an adult diaper on her was more than her dignity could handle.

As Art shared this story at his first counseling appointment, he wondered how he could continue to care for Delia at home. He was willing to do this out of love for her, but he also wanted to preserve her dignity. Art had hired a part-time caregiver, but since she wasn't there 24/7, Art still had to deal with Delia's toileting needs, and her resistance was getting worse. Tearfully, Art told Ed, "I feel that it's my duty to keep Delia at home. I'd be so ridden with guilt if I moved her into a facility I don't know if I could live with myself. We have long-term care insurance, but it won't cover around-the-clock caregivers, which one agency told me would cost $14,000 a month. My kids think Delia should go into the memory care unit at a facility just three miles from the house. They're worried about the toll full-time care partnering is taking on me."

On the Alzheimer's journey, one of the hardest decisions families face is the decision about placement in a long-term care facility. Many feel that placing their loved one in a facility amounts to abandonment. There are many reasons to consider facility placement, but most families face this decision because their loved one has reached the stage when assistance is needed with toileting, bathing, and dressing and/or there are inadequate financial resources to hire paid caregivers.

Family counseling is the most helpful way to facilitate the discussion and decision-making that surround the issue of facility placement. The initial family session, led by the involved medical or mental health provider, typically includes the spouse and adult children, but not the PWD. If one or more adult children live out of town, they can be included by phone, or via Skype or FaceTime.

Ed facilitated a family meeting for Art and his children. After this meeting the family decided to move Delia into a memory care unit in their town. Ed met with Art one year later. Art said, "I was full of uncertainty and guilt-ridden about the decision. Right after the move, I was deeply saddened about not sharing a bed with Delia any more, not having her around the house, knowing she'd never be back. But it became apparent very quickly that Delia's new environment was better for her. All of the agitation she had in reaction to me went away. I've learned that a one-hour visit, most days of the week, is best for both of us. We hug and kiss and play old songs that we both love. Sometimes we even dance. Our time together now is quality time.

"One of our favorite things is nap time. Delia rests her head on my shoulder; I hold her hand and tell her, 'I'm your husband;

you're my wife, and we're going to spend the rest of our lives together,' and she falls asleep. In retrospect, I realize that I had not fully accepted Delia's diagnosis, and the frustration and anger I felt inside was being passed along to Delia in my caregiving. I've now accepted that she has Alzheimer's, and the guilt has gone away. I know she's getting the best care possible."

A FAMILY MEETING AGENDA USUALLY INCLUDES:

1. A summary of where the patient currently is in their dementia journey and where they're headed next. A visual aid showing the stages of Alzheimer's disease (see chapter 4) helps establish a timeline.

2. A discussion of the diagnosis, prognosis, and care needs, with an opportunity for each family member to express their feelings, allowing the spouse to speak first.

3. A discussion of the available options, such as keeping the loved one at home versus placement in a facility, noting advantages and disadvantages, not just for the PWD, but also for each family member involved in their care.

4. An open discussion of how to stay connected and how to best love the family member with dementia, no matter what decision is made about where they will live.

Stories of *Hesed**

"Love bears up under anything and everything that comes . . . "
—1 Corinthians 13:7

TROY'S STORY: "SHE WAS TERRIFIED"

THE TAPESTRY OF A MARRIAGE relationship does not unravel overnight. It unravels slowly, just as it was woven, one conversation and one experience at a time. And, as Troy can attest, the unraveling can be as unnerving as it is inexplicable.

Troy met Danielle in 1986 when he took a job at the factory where she was working. Troy thought Danielle was, "the most beautiful woman I had ever laid eyes on." He was captivated by her smile and her "amazing blue eyes." As he got to know her, he was even more impressed by "how humble she was, and how helpful she was to everyone." More than anything, it was "her loving personality that caught my attention," he said.

At age 29, Danielle was eight and a half years older than Troy. Neither cared about the age difference though, and after dating for two years, they married. Danielle was the quiet introvert; Troy was "Mr. Outgoing, wanting to go and do whatever with anybody

Hesed: a Hebrew word that combines love and loyalty. It is not just a feeling but an action. *Hesed* is a merciful, intentional love that intervenes on behalf of loved ones and comes to their rescue.

to have fun." Their personality combination worked well, and in the early years of their marriage, Troy says, "We were best friends doing everything together." Then, inexplicably, when Danielle was 46 years old, she began to change.

Troy recalls the day he first noticed that something was amiss.

"We always did our own taxes," he said. "I came home from work one day and Danielle was on the bed with tax papers and receipts everywhere, just crying. And I said, 'What's wrong, Honey?' She looked at me through her tears and said, 'I can't do it. What's wrong with me? I can't do it.'"

Even more troubling, Troy began to notice that quiet, introverted Danielle was transforming into a defiant and argumentative woman he hardly recognized. She would yell, *"'You're not going to make me do this!'*—that kind of attitude," Troy recalled, "just vocal aggression." He was mystified. Prior to this, he said, "We'd agreed on pretty much everything." Worst of all, "Mr. Outgoing" now found himself married to Danielle the recluse.

"She wanted to stay home and didn't want *me* to go anywhere either. This was the biggest thing we used to argue over. It got to where she didn't want us to even go to the grocery store. She didn't want us to do *anything*.

"She would barricade us in our bedroom. She'd take the cord

of an electric heater and wrap it around the door handles and lock the door. She'd put stuff up against the windows. She shut the closet door and the bathroom door. Then she would hunker down in the bed. It's sad, but she was terrified."

Troy and Danielle sought help, but to no avail. Over a period of years, a laundry list of possible diagnoses accumulated: depression, menopause, stress, post-traumatic stress disorder, low sodium, pseudodementia, hormone problems, "she's making herself sick," and worst of all, "there's nothing wrong with her." All the while, said Troy, "her attitude and her reclusion were getting worse. She never wanted to leave our bedroom."

Finally, he had enough. He remembers thinking, "Well, if they are telling me she is fine and the medicines aren't helping, then I am not going to be a part of this."

"Her behavior was making me just have a loss of life," he said. "I didn't want to sit in a house, in my 30s, and not see anybody or do anything. It was driving me crazy. So I told her, 'I'm leaving, I'm not going to do this' and I moved out."

Troy checked on Danielle regularly and mowed the lawn for her, but they remained separated until one day, more than a year later, he finally learned the cause of Danielle's inexplicable behavior changes. When she was 52, a PET scan finally revealed Danielle's true diagnosis: early-onset Alzheimer's disease, now in the late stage. With this devastating diagnosis came a change of heart for Troy. He returned home to Danielle because he now understood that her disturbing behaviors were not really "her," but the disease that was taking hold of her. He said, "I came back because I realized what she was going through and what she was about to go through. Danielle wears it in her eyes, and I could see it: she was terrified. So I thought, 'She needs some support and strength and I am going to be there for her.'"

Troy now looks with regret upon the years that preceded Danielle's diagnosis. "There were some times in those years that I wasn't loving. I was hateful. I was very selfish," he admits. His decision to come back to Danielle, however, was the opposite of selfishness; it marked the beginning of an outpouring of *hesed* love upon Danielle that has continued from the spring of 2012 to the present. Today, those who know Troy are touched by his compassionate care of Danielle and his constant expressions of love to her. He is a role model for selfless, loving caregiving.

"Compassion is probably what has grown most in me because of what Danielle is suffering through," he said. "If there was any way I could take this disease from her, I would."

SANDRA'S STORY: "I AM NOT GOING TO ALLOW YOU TO TREAT HIM LIKE THAT"

"Work has always been a big part of my life," Sandra told us. Thirty years prior, a job offer from a major corporation had brought her to the city where she met Aaron, "a nice Jewish boy." They discovered that they were both "vineyard people" who also shared a love for foreign films, travel, and art. They married and had a son, Joel, and a daughter, Peyton.

"We had a fairly modern kind of independent marriage," Sandra said. "I did my thing and he did his." Throughout their marriage, though Sandra remained passionate about her career, the common interests she shared with Aaron created many opportunities for spending quality time together. Life was good.

When Aaron was 55 years old, Sandra realized that something about him had changed. Her guess was adult attention deficit disorder (ADD), and she encouraged him to see a doctor. "I thought I would just hear back about what pill he was on," she said, "but one appointment led to another." She wondered, "What are all these tests for?"

Aaron's worsening problem, whatever it was, began to strain the marriage. Sandra remembers, "It was a difficult time. There was friction. There was tension, but it really wasn't understood that it was something medical. There was a conscious pulling apart. I think on his end it was because he couldn't think, and on my end because I was disappointed in our interactions. We kind of went into our individual corners. It was deliberate on my part. I felt like his world was very narrow. I thought I would leave him."

We asked, "So what made you hang in there?"

She said, "Probably the kids."

Joel and Peyton, she said, also knew things were not right. "Their dad was not able to register it when they made a soccer goal. Sitting on the sidelines, he couldn't really celebrate, but none of us knew why," she said.

Unbeknownst to Sandra, Aaron was also experiencing serious difficulties at work. He couldn't remember his computer password. He was being assigned simpler tasks. Sandra later learned that coworkers were helping him and covering for him. Eventually, Aaron's employer presented him with a choice: resign or be fired. At age 57, after more than 30 years with the same employer, he resigned, still undiagnosed. Not long afterward, roughly two years after Sandra had first sent him in search of an ADD pill, the diagnosis came: early-onset Alzheimer's disease.

Sandra admitted, "In the beginning, I was kicking and screaming as a caregiver. It's not my *modus operandi*—I am not a caring, demonstrative kind of person. So, when we first got the diagnosis I was full throttle into finding places that could care for him or support groups that we could both go to. It was a chore. I was stressed. I felt very put upon and I just wanted to really get my career back on track. I am not proud of that; it's just how I was at the beginning of caregiving."

Then something very unexpected changed Sandra's attitude.

Weeks later, to relieve the stress of caregiving, Sandra took a weekend trip to New York City for some respite. She left Aaron at home in the care of professional male caregivers working in shifts. When Aaron woke up after a nap, two caregivers were present, and in a state of confusion, he hit one of them. He would not stop hitting, so they called for assistance, which resulted in his being transported to a hospital emergency room. In the ER things went from bad to worse. He hit a nurse and was placed in restraints. When he pulled the restraints off, the security staff got involved. Aaron somehow ended up with a black eye and a severe abrasion on his arm.

Sandra had been contacted and arrived at the ER a few hours later. The attending physician urged her to involuntarily commit Aaron, but could not tell her where he would be placed. In that moment, Sandra said, "It became very clear that the rest of the world wasn't going to care for him. He was tethering out of reality. I literally pulled him back and brought him home. The doctor was afraid that he was going to be violent. I didn't know what I had on my hands. I just knew that what was happening in the ER was untenable."

That experience, said Sandra, "was a turning point for me. I went from being a reluctant caregiver to being full-in. I kind of circled the wagons. Aaron was physically and mentally wounded and I became his adamant protector. I became fully involved in a very deliberate way: 'You are not going to do this to him. I am not going to allow you to treat him like that.' In this crisis I learned how much I did love him," she said. "I became instinctive—all-in and total care, total focus, and trying to get him back on track."

Aaron lived just 70 days after the ER incident. During those 10 weeks, despite his unusually rapid decline, Sandra's impassioned "all-in" focus allowed their love to be surprisingly and beautifully rekindled. She reached out to Aaron with all five love languages during this time.

"We had not ever given each other a lot of gifts," she said, "but I would say that my gift to him after the crisis was just time and singular focus." At home, Sandra would sit with him and watch TV. Outside their home, she intentionally focused on the things they had enjoyed from the beginning of their relationship.

"We carried on as long as we could, doing things that we like to do. I took him to vineyards probably past where other people would have been comfortable doing that. We went to a movie, and the movie in particular was awkward, but I continued our *Quality Time* until the end. Because even if there were awkward things or weird things, the positive outweighed some of the negative.

"Before the crisis, there weren't a lot of *Words of Affirmation*," Sandra said. "At the very end, when he was so lacking in capability, in the morning if he got himself through toileting, I would say, 'This is fantastic!' It was just like parenting an 18-month-old, and in his 18-month-old world, I was affirming. He was in a very different space from his full manhood. Sometimes he would say, 'Don't talk to me about this.' He wasn't happy to be receiving affirmation at the level where he was, but other times he would say, "Yeah, this is great. I did do great."

"*Physical Touch* got reintroduced after the crisis," she said. "After he got out of the ER in such bad shape, he needed my hand to steady him and for reassurance, and touch became a very strong connector. We have a convertible and I would take him on long rides and we would hold hands, which we hadn't done in years. He was capable of talking until the very end. But there wasn't a need for him to talk because it was just an unencumbered kind of drive. Touch became important at movies too; he was just happy holding hands. After the ER experience, he was fighting sleep. So, I would lie down with him and hold his hand, which I didn't do before. He was very happy when I held his hand.

"He was able at various times to say how grateful he was. That was not typical. It was often when I was holding his hand and accompanying him to the bathroom and onto the toilet. He understood that I was the link to him being able to function and survive. He said, 'Thank you, I love you. You're the best.' And it was in the midst of hand holding, usually en route to getting him to where he needed to be, that he expressed those words.

"The night before he died, he told me he loved me. We had been mostly holding hands for two hours. And I think somehow he knew that he was not much longer for this world. He said he loved me and he kissed me on my lips, which was not usual."

Looking back, Sandra said, "As horrible as the ER experience was, it gave us an opportunity to create a love connection that had not been as strong prior to this crisis."

THE EMPATHY OF *HESED*

For a long time, neither Troy nor Sandra could fathom a reason for the odd and hurtful behaviors of their spouses. Both concluded that their marriages were doomed. Troy actually left, and Sandra was contemplating her exit. What brought Troy back and what kept Sandra from leaving was their compassionate realization that their spouses were helpless in the throes of the disease that had gripped their lives.

In *The 5 Love Languages®*, Gary wrote, "Encouragement requires empathy and seeing the world from your spouse's perspective."[1] For both Troy and Sandra, suddenly seeing the world from the perspective of their spouse was a wake-up call that changed their attitudes. Both decided to remain married and to lovingly support their spouses as they struggled through their dementia journey. As Gary wrote, "love is always a choice."[2] Both Troy and Sandra did a U-turn because they chose to love unselfishly: *hesed.*

JON'S STORY: "WHO'S THAT MAN IN THE CAR?"

Lewy Body Dementia

About Lewy Body Dementia:[3] *Until now, we have focused mainly on Alzheimer's disease because, as mentioned in chapter 1, it is the most common type of dementia, accounting for 60–80 percent of all dementia cases. Far fewer people have ever heard of Lewy body dementia (LBD), the third most common type of dementia, affecting between 1 and 1.4 million people in the United States. (Vascular dementia, usually caused by strokes, is second.)*

LBD is an umbrella term for several forms of dementia that result from the presence of Lewy bodies (abnormal protein deposits) in the brain. Far more men than women get LBD. Because LBD is not as common as Alzheimer's, LBD patients, care partners and family members often have difficulty obtaining an accurate diagnosis and finding peer support. (For more information about LBD, see "Non-Alzheimer's Dementias" in Appendix B.)

Jon and Suzanne met in 1969 when they were both university students. They had noticed each other at fraternity parties but had not actually met. Jon said, "It turned out that we were living in the same apartment building. She was on the third floor and I was on the second." They discovered their common residence one warm summer day when Suzanne was taking out the trash. Jon recalled, "She was bringing her garbage out through the back stairs, and it's kind of hilarious. She had on a tank top and shorts and she carried the bag in front of her. When I saw her coming down the stairs, all I saw was bare-skin little arms and bare-skin legs. And her eyes. She was gorgeous. I thought, 'Man, that's an attractive girl.' She saw me and said 'Hi.' I realized that I had seen her at parties and so we started getting together."

"It was a love affair from the beginning," he said. "She was just a perfect fit for me. She was very energetic, loved to explore, and was creative. We had this playful thing going on between us all of our lives together, before marriage and after."

After college, they married, had two children, and enjoyed successful careers, which took them to three different cities over the course of their marriage. "In every neighborhood that we moved into," said Jon, "Suzanne would form some sort of party group. Something was always going on at our house. She loved costumes and dressing up, and dressing up the kids. Parties for the kids were outrageously fun. And there were spontaneous parties. We were a magnet for other couples like us. We always had a group of people that enjoyed board games, charades, Pictionary, parties, all that kind of stuff. We sought them out, but they sought us out too. It made life so wonderful because Suzanne's personality was just so complementary to mine.

"We enjoyed each other's company so much that we tended

to do a lot of things together. We had our separate lives, her teaching and my work, which involved some travel. But around the house, yard work, cooking, evenings, it was our time. It was very, very good. It was just a wonderful life," he said.

In 2009, Jon began to notice certain oddities in Suzanne's behavior. He said, "She would ask me for coffee when it was right in front of her." I would point that out and she would say, 'Oh' and she would look at it." She became confused about "the simplest things," he said, like "how to use an ice maker on the refrigerator door, forgetting that you have to push, you can't just hold your cup there."

He knew Suzanne was experiencing what she thought were anxiety attacks and that she had sought treatment for this from a psychiatrist. What he didn't know was "that she had given up driving," he said. "She was walking places during the day while I was at work."

In 2010, Suzanne, a very accomplished photographer, began to ask questions of fellow photography club members that they found concerning. One asked Jon, "Is Suzanne okay? She is acting like she doesn't understand her camera." Jon said, "I was also noticing that she couldn't button up correctly. And if I was holding a jacket for her, she would find one arm, but no matter what I did, she couldn't find the other. So, I would have her put both arms behind her and I would slip both arms on at the same time. The ability to do sequential tasks was the next thing that she lost—the ability to do step 1, 2, and 3. That concerned me."

The watershed event occurred in July of 2011. "Suzanne went on a cruise with five of her childhood friends that got together annually. I thought if anything grounded her, it would be these five friends," Jon said. "While they were at sea I got a message from their cruise ship. Her friends were concerned because she suddenly didn't recognize them. She had been acting anxious and wary and she finally said to one of them, "Who are you and what are we doing here?"

Jon told Suzanne's psychiatrist about the cruise ship incident. He ordered tests which, Jon said, "demonstrated impairment in lots of areas." The psychologist that tested her used the words, "severely impaired," and told Jon, "Do not leave her alone at home." In September, at the age of 61, Suzanne was diagnosed with Lewy body dementia. Jon immediately retired from his job and turned his full attention to her care.

He recalled, "One day, Suzanne cautiously said to me, 'Could you call Patty?', (a friend of ours), so I made the call. Suzanne got on the phone and whispered, 'Can I come over?' and Patty said, 'Sure.' I drove her to Patty's house and when we parked, Suzanne quickly got out of the car and rushed to the front door. She asked Patty, 'Who's in the car? Who's that man in the car?' Patty reassured her that it was Jon, her husband."

"It got increasingly worse," he said. "Almost daily, she would give me that look of, 'I don't know who you are. Why are you in my house?' During a conversation with her sister-in-law, Suzanne suddenly leaned forward and said, 'Will you tell me where Jon is?' Her sister-in-law responded, 'He is right there.' Suzanne exclaimed, 'Why is everyone doing this? Why won't anyone tell me? What is going on here? Where is he?'" From that point on, Jon said, "She didn't know me as her husband."

"The husband-and-wife relationship was tricky territory for several months in 2013, trying to figure out how we could relate," he said. "Touching, kissing on the cheek, hugging, any kind of touch would make her anxious. And she would say things like,

'Are you the manager? Who pays you?' She was thinking of me as the facility manager at a place that she was living. If I exited to take a shower and change clothes, and then re-entered the room, she might say, 'There you are!' Then 30 seconds or a minute or two later, she would go back to, 'No you're not.' She would say 'Oh, there you are!' in the way you would say it if you hadn't seen a friend in years and suddenly you bumped into them at the market. Just a delighted type of excitement. Then she would lapse back into, 'Well, that's the other Jon.'"

For the duration of her illness, Suzanne continued to believe that Jon was not her husband, but a lookalike impostor. This delusion, known as Capgras syndrome, affects approximately 17 percent of people with LBD, according to a study cited by the Lewy Body Dementia Association.[4] (As mentioned in chapter 3, Capgras syndrome can also occur in AD.)

Jon said, "I was told by a therapist that I should not confront the delusion nor confirm it. I had to basically consider our relationship as she did, a 'kindness of strangers' type thing. The best I could get after 2012 was just a comfortable friendship. She was very thankful for the kindness of the stranger named Jon."

> "Early in the disease I was fighting it, saying, 'I am going to convince her that I am Jon.'"

Though Suzanne never again recognized Jon as her husband, his love for her never waned, though his heart was breaking. He would watch helplessly as Suzanne walked around the house crying, "Where's Jon? Why am I left alone? Is he coming back?" He said, "Almost every day, numerous times, I desperately wanted to cover her hands in mine and say, 'I love you.' But, it would frighten her. Because to her, I was Jon, the manager of the facility, or Jon, the kindly guide taking her to doctors' appointments. Early in the disease I was fighting it, saying, 'I am going to convince her that I am Jon.' But if I touched her shoulders I could see that I wasn't giving her peace; I was giving her anxiety.

"One day I was in the bedroom, changing the sheets on her bed, and she came up behind me and threw a box of tissues and hit me in the back. She demanded, 'Look at me!' I turned around and she said, 'Why won't you tell me where Jon is?' And I just had given up at that point on trying to answer," he said.

In his role as "kind stranger," Jon tried to maintain normalcy, continuing to do ordinary things with Suzanne. He recalled, "Once at a coffee shop, she was at the counter and she wanted to put a sugar in her coffee. The barista gave her the coffee and said, 'The sugar is behind you.' So, she turned around but she didn't process what he had said. She turned back to him and said, 'Can I have some sugar?' He said, 'It is behind you.' She just stood there. Then he got frustrated. He said, really loud, and in front of others, 'LADY, IT'S RIGHT THERE!' She just set her coffee down and left. I was there with her and I said, 'No, no, no,' and I got her coffee and I got the sugar. Those types of experiences were just devastating to her. She just didn't want to go back. She started slowly withdrawing and she eventually became unable to go anyplace, even for a simple drive. Her brain was just not processing the world."

For most people with Lewy body dementia, insight is typically preserved. In that sense, Suzanne was typical, and remained, in Jon's words, "very perceptive." She always knew that something was terribly wrong and she tried desperately to get herself back on track. Jon recalled, "She would just plead with me, 'Would you please help me? Somebody has got to help me. Maybe, can you take me to the doctor?'" Near the end of her life, he said, "I found pieces of paper where she had written her name, my name, the kids' names again and again. And she would rehearse her own name out loud over and over: 'Suzanne Griffin, Suzanne Griffin, Suzanne Griffin.' Like a person hanging on the edge of a cliff, she was trying to hang on, I think."

From the time he began caring for her, Jon's focus was on loving and comforting Suzanne in every way possible. After the LBD diagnosis and his hasty retirement, he sold their home and built a new one closer to their daughter and grandchildren, believing this new home would be more comfortable for Suzanne. When she no longer recognized him as her husband, he hired caregivers and moved into a separate bedroom. Early in the disease, she would allow him to give her foot rubs and would accept little trinkets as gifts. Later, he made sure she ate and administered her medicines and washed her hair. There were daily drives in the car, listening to music, arm massages, and repositioning her bed so she could see out the window. "Whatever calmed her, I would do. I would just drop everything and do it," he said.

On January 27, 2015, Suzanne fell and broke her hip. That day Jon made a decision: he would say the words, 'I love you.' "I said it a hundred times a day," he said. "I decided that even if it made her anxious, it was better that she hear it: 'I love you. I love you. I love you. You are loved. Your children love you. Your grandchildren love you. I love you—Jon loves you.' I said it just constantly."

On the last Sunday of her life, Suzanne entered a hospice care facility. The hospice staff wanted to give her a bed bath and a shampoo. As they pulled the privacy curtain around her, Suzanne cried out, "Jon!" It was the last time she spoke. The following Wednesday morning, just after sunrise, Suzanne passed away, her hand in the hand of her loving husband of 40 years.

"My kindest friends encourage me by saying how blessed I was and how our marriage was unique," he said. "Our life was rich and full and many couples don't have that." Recalling her relentless pursuit of the "real" Jon throughout her illness, he reflected tenderly, "It told me that she loved me immensely. Her anguish was proportionate to her love."

GRACIE'S STORY: "I AM MARRIED BUT LIVE ALONE"

Frontotemporal Dementia

About Frontotemporal Dementia (FTD):[5,6,7] *Frontotemporal dementia is an umbrella term for conditions that cause portions of the frontal and temporal lobes of the brain to shrink and lose function. These lobes govern behavior, language, personality, and physical movement. The most common signs and symptoms of FTD are extreme behavior and personality changes. People with the disease may become impulsive, rude, emotionally indifferent, and apt to behave in socially inappropriate ways, without the insight to recognize that their words and behaviors are offensive.*

FTD, the fourth most common type of dementia, may account for up to 10 percent of all dementia cases, affecting an estimated 140,000– 350,000 people in the US. Unlike AD, which becomes more likely as people age, FTD typically affects younger people. Among those younger than age 65, FTD is the most common dementia after early-onset AD. Because FTD is far less common than Alzheimer's disease, as with

Lewy body dementia, FTD patients and family members often have difficulty obtaining an accurate diagnosis and finding peer support. (For more information about FTD, see "Non-Alzheimer's Dementias" in Appendix B.)

Gracie met Ken when she was just 17 years old. Her best friend introduced them and Ken called Gracie the very next day to ask her out. She accepted his invitation—she thought—for the next Saturday night. But when he called midweek to confirm a pickup time for Friday, she realized her mistake.

"I thought you said Saturday. I have a date for Friday."

"I have a date for Saturday," he said. "Tell you what. If you break your date, I'll break mine, and I'll take you out both nights."

Said Gracie, "Fifty years later, here we are."

"He was cute," she recalled, but more importantly, "he was kind. I just loved that kindness. I had never been treated kindly before."

Growing up with an angry, alcoholic father, Gracie couldn't help but notice that Ken's family life was different. She said, "Ken embraced family and I had never seen that before. He was loyal to his family, respectful to them, and he was fun. He had so many admirable qualities. He was humorous. Always a hard worker. I didn't just love him, I loved his family. They were gentle. They were respectful and kind. I just loved their calmness."

She recalled a long-ago Sunday afternoon. "We were kids. We were in college and we had two more years and we wanted to get married. Ken was outside talking to his dad, and his mother and I were in the house. His mom said, 'You know what he's doing out there with his dad, don't you?' I said no. She said, 'Well, he's talking to his dad about how we might help you finance school if you want to get married. You better get out there and help him!'"

Excited, she went outside and joined in the conversation. She can still vividly remember Ken's father sitting in an old-fashioned, green porch swing talking with them about the future they envisioned as husband and wife.

With nostalgia in her voice, Gracie said, "We were just back on the farm where Ken grew up this past weekend. His brother's widow lives there now. Ken and I sat in that same swing."

Did he remember the swing?

"Oh yes. He remembered. I said, 'Your daddy was sitting in this swing when we were talking to him about getting married.' We courted in that swing. I rocked my babies in that swing. His mother and I snapped beans together sitting in that swing. So, that swing, oh my gosh, that swing is who we are. It's such a beautiful symbol. It is just precious to me. I cried. It didn't mean a thing to Ken. He felt nothing being with me in that swing."

Through the years, the old farmhouse porch swing has changed very little. ("It's still the same color. They keep it painted green.") Ken, however, has changed greatly.

"We married very young, 20 and 21," Gracie said. "We always had a great marriage. Always had a great intimate relationship, touching, hugging, watching TV and holding hands. Ken was fun. We would fish together and boat together. We had a river place for 10 years of our marriage. We both loved the water. I loved that we had a lot of common interests."

They had two children. Over the years they bought ten old houses and lived in each one while they remodeled

> "I have decided that I will never touch you again."

it together, then "flipped it" for a profit and moved on to the next one. Then, in the midst of so much happiness, inexplicably, Ken began to pull away from Gracie.

She pleaded with him, "What is happening? I don't understand it."

He told her, "In 1974 you said something to my mother that was very unkind, and I have just decided that I am going to punish you for that. I'm not going to forgive you."

She said, "Ken, that makes no sense. Your mom and I are best friends."

Weeks later things were no better. Mystified, Gracie remembers saying, "Look, Ken, what is wrong?" He responded, "Well, I remember one time you said I was only interested in you for sex, so I have decided that I will never touch you again."

Gracie knew they needed help. She said, "We went to a marriage counselor. The first time he met with us, he said, 'What seems to be the problem?' Ken said, 'I don't have a problem. She does.'" Not surprisingly, counseling failed. (The counselor actually quit in the middle of their third session, telling them, "I think you're wasting my time and your money.")

The gulf between them continued to widen, no matter how Gracie tried to repair the breach. Ken, said Gracie, was "argumentative, argumentative, argumentative." She said, "He got fired from three jobs because he challenged the boss." For more than a decade, she struggled to understand what had happened to the fun and satisfying marriage they once had. Year after year, she said, "the arguing was a problem, disrespect for authority was a problem, the loss of jobs was a problem, intimacy was a problem, and he began to spend more and more time by himself. He 'left' me about 12 years ago.

"About three years ago I finally said, 'We are going to the doctor. We're going to prove, one way or the other, that one of us has an issue. If it turns out that we don't, then this will just be how our marriage ended up, and we need to be thinking about where we are going with this marriage. But, if one of us has a problem, we can get help.' Ken told her, 'I'll go because I'm going to prove it's you.'"

Initial testing seemed to indicate that Ken was in the beginning stage of Alzheimer's disease. Then about a year and a half ago, a geriatrician specializing in dementia diagnosis told Ken, "You do not have Alzheimer's disease. I'm not sure what this is yet, so we are going to do more testing."

"They did a PET scan, which was read by two experts," Gracie said. "The doctor called me shortly thereafter and said, 'I am going to give you a clinical diagnosis of frontotemporal dementia.' I had never heard of this. I started researching FTD. Now it all makes sense. Looking back, I've had so many aha moments— so *that's* what it was!"

For more than a decade, Gracie had no explanation for the radical changes in Ken's behavior. Learning his diagnosis finally gave Gracie the *why* she had so earnestly sought. Unfortunately, understanding the illness has not improved their marriage or taken away her gnawing sense of loneliness. Since the day 12 years ago when Ken told her, "I will never touch you again," he has remained physically and emotionally isolated from her.

"He has a little 'man cave' out in the garage area with a TV, fridge, and air conditioner. So he spends his whole day by himself. He does come into the house for dinner, which he eats in front of the TV. He does not talk. After dinner he goes back to the man cave. He comes to bed around 1:00 or 2:00 a.m. When he gets in bed," Gracie said, "he always turns his back to me."

"I am married," she said, "but I live alone. I do not have a life partner. He's not really interested in my job. We don't talk about the future. We don't talk about buying a new couch. We don't talk about anything."

Gracie noted a painful irony: Ken seems to want to touch everyone but her. Happily, he does still hug his adult children and grandchildren. Not so happily, he imposes unwanted hugs upon strangers in the grocery store and male clerks in home-improvement stores. At the doctor's office, he puts his arms around the staff. On occasion he has also put his arms around women he did not know and made sexually suggestive comments to them. FTD has robbed him of the insight to know that his behavior is socially inappropriate and embarrassing to his family. He does not recognize that his life and his marriage have been altered by FTD. Gracie said that when she loses patience with him, "He laughs and tells me, 'I don't have a disease. You are the crazy one.'"

> "I want him to be accountable, knowing he can't be accountable."

After so many years of emotional and physical estrangement from her husband, Gracie's emotional love tank is nearly bone-dry—at most, she says, "one, on a scale of one to ten."

"Before I knew the diagnosis, I felt anger and hate toward Ken. Lots of disrespect for him. Since the diagnosis," she admitted, "I still feel some anger. I still want to blame him, even though I know I can't blame him. I want him to be accountable for some stuff, knowing that he can't be accountable."

THE EXPERIMENT

In *The 5 Love Languages*®, Gary recounted the story of a woman named Ann who felt much the same as Gracie.[8] Her emotional tank was empty and her marriage was painful. Others had told her the same thing Gracie has been told: it's hopeless; leave him. Ann's response was the same as Gracie's has been: "I just can't bring myself to do that."

Feeling trapped between the proverbial "rock and a hard place," Ann said, "Dr. Chapman, I just don't know if I can ever love him again after all he has done to me."

Gary told her, "I am deeply sympathetic with your struggle. You are in a very difficult situation. I wish I could offer you an easy answer. Unfortunately, I can't." However, knowing she was a woman of deep personal faith, an idea occurred to him.

Here is an excerpt from the book:

> "I want to read something that Jesus once said that I think has some application to your marriage." I read slowly and deliberately.
>
> *"But to you who are listening I say: Love your enemies, do good to those who hate you, bless those who curse you, pray for those who mistreat you. . . . Do to others as you would have them do to you . . . "*
>
> "Does that sound like your husband? Has he treated you as an enemy rather than as a friend?"
>
> She paused. "Yes," she said quietly.
>
> "Has he ever cursed you?" I asked.
>
> "Many times."

"Has he ever mistreated you?"

"Often."

"And has he told you that he hates you?"

"Yes."

"Ann, if you are willing, I would like to do an experiment. I would like to see what would happen if we apply this principle to your marriage. Let me explain what I mean." I went on to explain to Ann the concept of the emotional tank and the fact that when the tank is low, as hers was, we have no love feelings toward our spouse but simply experience emptiness and pain . . . "Certainly we do not have warm feelings for people who hate us. That would be abnormal, but we can do loving acts for them. That is simply a choice. We hope that such loving acts will have a positive effect upon their attitudes and behavior and treatment, but at least we have chosen to do something positive for them."

Though it was extremely difficult, Ann began to consistently reach out to her husband, Glenn, with the love languages. Over the next six months, she saw a tremendous change in Glenn's attitude and treatment of her. Amazingly, the marriage was repaired.

Gary wrote, "To this day, Glenn swears to his friends that I am a miracle worker. I know in fact that love is a miracle worker. Perhaps you need a miracle in your own marriage. Why not try Ann's experiment?"

When we interviewed Gracie for this book, the parallels between Ann's situation and hers were obvious. The difference, however, was stark: Ann's husband was cognitively normal; Gracie's husband has a type of dementia that creates emotional indifference and impairs both empathy and insight. Given this, could Ann's experiment possibly succeed for Gracie too? We challenged Gracie to give it a try. Though she was "very hurt about the way Ken had treated me," she agreed to try the experiment anyway. We reminded her that she had absolutely nothing to lose.

Gracie recalled, "I went into it with a negative attitude, expecting nothing, or very little if he did happen to respond. I was playing the role of the 'victim,' which is easy to do with this disease." Nonetheless, Gracie began to deliberately show love to Ken. She served him meals, brought treats to him in the "man cave," snuggled up to him in bed, and spoke affirming words to him. All of these kindnesses were met with indifference or resistance. She kept a journal, noting everything she did, how she felt about it, and how Ken reacted.

Within a few days, there was a change—but not with Ken.

"This is where it gets really amazing," she said. "After the first couple of days, I would reread the previous journal entries stating all my acts of service, from making his morning coffee to taking a late night snack to the 'man cave' before I went to bed. I began to realize, *This is what God does for me every single day and I am not required to acknowledge His gifts. He gives gifts just because He loves me. That's all: He loves me.* I have loved Ken since I was 18 years old and it dawned on me that now I was making it a *conditional* love: if Ken responds, then I will do acts of service for him again; if he does not, then I pull away. I began to get so excited about showing Ken *unconditional* love, and he is not required to acknowledge one thing. I began to do these kindnesses for my pleasure and to honor God. I started to have fun with it.

"Now I look for things in the grocery store that I know he

would like, special cookies or candies. Every day I offer to take him anywhere he needs to go. I speak kind words to him often, and most of the time he does not respond and just leaves the room. But the 'experiment' is no longer about seeing if Ken will express love back to me. It has become about what can I do for him that honors him, and therefore honors God. I once again see the young man I fell in love with, the man who was so faithful to his family for so many years. I am still devastated that he has this terrible disease, but I understand more each day the vows of 'till death do us part.' As I keep choosing to go into Ken's world, doing these acts of serving and saying kind words gives me pleasure and joy.

"During the weeks I have been doing this experiment, there have been three little responses from Ken. Once I was at the sink and he walked up to me and gave me a peck on the cheek and walked away. That's it. But it was HUGE for me—he has not kissed me in many, many years. Once, he leaned in towards me to *almost* give me a hug. There was no physical touch, but I called it a hug! Then, we had a burger at a neighborhood place the week of Valentine's Day. Two days later he asked me if I had enjoyed the dinner. I said, 'Yes. I like going there.' He said, 'Great! Happy Valentine's.'"

Although the experiment we asked Gracie to try is now finished, she does not plan to stop speaking the five love languages to Ken, even if he makes no further response. We wondered, would she encourage others to try the same experiment?

She said, "It is like you all told me: 'What have you got to lose?' So yes, I would encourage others to do this, first learning the loved one's Love Language and then responding with that on a daily basis. I believe we as care partners have the ability to do more for our loved ones than any doctor, medicine, or counseling. We have the ability to try to reach them in a way that science knows little about—speaking to their love language. Although some days may be harder than others, I promise it will be a success, either for the patient, the care partner, or hopefully both, and in ways you probably never imagined."

7

Voices of Experience

"Experience is not what happens to you;
it's what you do with what happens to you."
–ALDOUS HUXLEY

WE INVITED EIGHT VETERAN dementia care partners to participate in a focus group. In preparation for the meeting, we shared information with them about the five love languages and asked them to take the love languages quiz, once for themselves, and once on behalf of the spouse for whom they provide care. In addition, because most of their spouses are in the middle or late stage of Alzheimer's disease, we asked them to answer the three questions that appear with the quizzes in chapter 2. We instructed them to combine this information and take their best guess at their spouse's pre-dementia love language. We also called their attention to *hesed* love, defining it for them as we did in chapter 2, a love that:

- acts out of unswerving loyalty
- can be counted on

- is not about the thrill of romance, but the security of faithfulness
- intervenes on behalf of loved ones and comes to their rescue

We told them, "As veteran care partners whose opinions we greatly value, today you are joining us as coauthors."

Our focus group participants were:

Penny, married for 34 years to Dennis (diagnosis: Alzheimer's disease) and his care partner for 7 years. Love languages—Penny: *Acts of Service*; Dennis: *Physical Touch*

Troy, married for 29 years to Danielle (diagnosis: early-onset Alzheimer's disease) and her care partner for 9 years. Love languages—Troy: *Quality Time*; Danielle: *Quality Time*

Allen, married for 57 years to Daisy (diagnosis: Alzheimer's disease) and her care partner for 3 years. Love languages—Allen: *Words of Affirmation*; Daisy: *Quality Time*

JoAnne, married for 45 years to Jerry (diagnosis: frontotemporal dementia) and his care partner for 2 ½ years. Love languages—JoAnne: *Acts of Service*; Jerry: *Gifts*

Betsy, married for 38 years to Brent (diagnosis: Alzheimer's disease) and his care partner for 10 years. Love languages—Betsy: *Words of Affirmation*; Brent: *Quality Time*

Angela, married for 35 years to Henry (diagnosis: early-onset Alzheimer's disease) and his care partner for 2 years. Love languages—Angela: *Acts of Service*; Henry: *Words of Affirmation*

Rick, married for 10 years to Stephanie (diagnosis: Alzheimer's disease) and her care partner for 5 years. Love languages—Rick: *Acts of Service*; Stephanie: *Acts of Service*

Sarah, married for 55 years to Bob (diagnosis: Alzheimer's disease) and his care partner for 6 years. Love languages—Sarah: *Acts of Service*; Bob: *Acts of Service*

As we had hoped, the group's hour and a half conversation yielded many valuable, heartfelt insights into the caregiving experience. Although we "primed the pump" with a few questions, we mostly listened, allowing the conversation to flow naturally, touching on a range of topics. Some participants' comments, unknown to them, mirrored key points from chapters we had already written. Other comments were pearls of wisdom that could only have been spoken by such experienced care partners. There were moments of laughter as well as tears as the group both affirmed each other's caregiving efforts and offered their seasoned advice for readers on the caregiving journey.

Below, we have excerpted portions of the audio transcript, grouping comments by topic. In a few places we have added our own comments or reflections.

"I PICK MYSELF BACK UP": WHAT THEY TOLD US

Lessons Learned

Penny: I say to myself each day, "You need to remember, old girl, that it is harder being a 75-year-old toddler than being the caregiver of a 75-year-old toddler."

Sarah: Early on I used to argue with Bob. I found out that's not such a good idea. You have to pick your battles. Now, if he says, "It's blue" and it's really green, I say, "Yes, it's blue."

Angela: I have learned that you have to grieve each change. I just have to have some days of sadness, but I know I can't stay on

> "One thing I wish I had learned sooner is that Brent can't remember that he can't remember." —BETSY

that path. I grieve the new loss and then I pick myself back up and move on to do and be what my husband needs.

Allen: It took me a while to learn that instead of raising my voice at Daisy because she couldn't find something, I should just back out of the room and have a little word with myself. I don't talk to myself much, but it works really well!

Betsy: One thing I wish I had learned sooner is that Brent can't remember that he can't remember. If I'd had that ingrained in me years ago, maybe I wouldn't have had health problems, the frustration, and the anger. But it's just hard to keep that in your brain 24/7/365. And if you just realize that sooner rather than later, I think it would be helpful.

Dementia Changes Everything

Rick: There's no point in trying to reason with your loved one. There's no point in saying, "Do you realize how irritating that is?" or "Could you not have expressed that better?" "Could you not be more appreciative?" There's no point in saying any of that. All that logic has long since gone out the window.

Penny: It changes the relationship in ways that are very difficult to describe. There are so many ironies. One is, at the very time when the care partner needs to do everything, the person for whom you care really does need more time and more touch and more of the things that don't get the tasks of life done.

Sarah: Even though my husband is showing all this love, he's just a different person now. He's not the one that I married 55 years ago.

If You're Sick, They're Sick

Sarah: If we have a conversation it always comes back to him. If I say, "I don't feel good today" or "This is hurting today," he says, "yes, mine hurts like that, too." Everything that I say, he reflects.

Troy: If you're in a bad mood or you're sick, they're sick. So you've got to focus your attention always on being upbeat and happy and loving, because then they feel that. Danielle does.

Rick: I love what you mentioned, that if there is something wrong with yourself, they always turn it around. If I say, "Gosh, I have a headache," first you get a little bit of a concern: "What's wrong? What do you think the matter is? Is it serious?"

"No, no, Honey, it's not serious."

"Well, I think I know just how you feel because I had a headache earlier."

Penny: Some of Dennis's female problems are getting worse! (*Laughter from the group.*) If you don't have a sense of humor, you're just not going to make it.

"Parent-Child"

Rick: It really is like taking care of a child, a child who is perpetually sick and you don't get any breaks.

Penny: The parent/child relationship is what it feels like to me. Early in this journey, Dennis was trying to express to someone how much he appreciated all that I was doing for him and he said, "She's like my mother. She takes care of everything." He meant that in the most wonderful way possible. But—I'll just say it—it ran up me like a streak of lightning. Then when he becomes frustrated or angry because I'm trying to help him with what needs to be done at that moment, it turns around the other way: "You're not my mother!" So you get it going and coming.

Betsy: I think as this journey progresses, that gets harder for me because I feel sometimes like I'm hugging my child and it's just weird.

Rick: Stephanie was only approaching 50 when she was diagnosed and we very, very quickly went into "parent/child" mode and physical intimacy seemed to go out the window. I tried to get closer, like in bed. Usually I'm on one side of the bed and she's on the other, and I tried to be more intimate. I tried to hold her longer and she really found it uncomfortable.

"A Part of You Dies with Them Each Day"

Allen: Since I retired eight years ago, I'm doing things I never thought about doing and doing things that Daisy always did diligently. It's just a whole cycle, 360 degrees, changing your life to be a care partner. It is really a long day sometimes, doing the things you have to do. For example, now to go to bed, it probably takes us 30 minutes to take the trousers off, or the dress off, or whatever. It's a real change in your life and you just have to adapt to it.

Rick: One of the greatest problems is anticipatory grief. You know that it's not going to end well, and every so often that just hits you. You have good times and you have really bad times, but always on your shoulder is this idea that there is a great sadness ahead of you and there's no getting around it.

Sarah: It's such a different kind of love that you give to the loved one. A part of you dies with them each day, and it's hard; it's hard.

Rick: In our hierarchy of needs, there's not much opportunity for the upper-level needs to be met. It's all just basic life-giving to our loved one. It's what we did for our children. There is not room there for play; there's not room there for joy. It's all lower-level hierarchy of need-type things. The joy and the fun, there are slight opportunities, but not a lot of opportunities for those things. So much of the color has gone out of my life.

> "You know that it's not going to end well, and every so often that just hits you." —RICK

Giving and Receiving Love Via the Five Love Languages

Betsy: One thing that keeps coming back to me is, as care partners we have to determine what their love language is at every point. It changes. The *Acts of Service* and *Quality Time* and all of that may not have been what they needed before this hit, but now we have to be receptive in the moment: what is their love language *right now?* You just have to, in the moment, ask, "What do they need us to do to show our love for them?" because it changes.

JoAnne: *Quality Time* is a little different now. We do still like to just be together. It's not a big deal just being together, but there's not very much conversation now. It's hard to have a back and forth: "What do you think about this? What do you think about that?" That's gone, but he still sits with me in the evening and we watch the news, *Wheel of Fortune*, and *Jeopardy.*

Angela: My love language is *Acts of Service* and my husband, through the years, has always been great at taking care of me, doing things for me just to make life easier for me. And he's still my husband in early-onset Alzheimer's and he still realizes that what I need is *Acts of Service*, but his acts of service look a little bit different now. He'll say, "I will empty the dishwasher for you," and he can't find his way around in the kitchen. He empties the dishwasher and he puts things all different places, everywhere, and when I need it, I'm searching the kitchen for where he's put it. But I just accept that act of service to me. I don't say, "You put it in the wrong place."

One day I wasn't feeling well, but I was vacuuming and he said, "You don't feel good. Let me do that." And I realized he doesn't know how to vacuum anymore. He took the vacuum cleaner and he pushed it around in a circle and he said, "There, the floor is vacuumed. You can rest now." But it's still very meaningful to me. Though it may look different, he is still showing me *Acts of Service* and acts of love that he can still do for me.

Penny: *Acts of Service* is a natural part of who I am. I think that's been true my whole life. And yet, as much as that's in my DNA, it's amazing that it can sometimes get really hard to enjoy being your natural self with the person you most want to serve. And one of the inner struggles, if I'm honest with myself, is that sometimes I just try to go numb and that makes being of help harder for me. I wonder what it feels like to him, how he might sense that, and that adds a layer of guilt.

Allen: Daisy will come up to me and just look at me and say, "Thank you. Thank you for taking such good care of me." *(Note: this is very meaningful to Allen because Daisy is speaking his primary love language, Words of Affirmation.)*

Relational Intimacy

Rick: Any time Stephanie thanks me for anything, I thank her back. Or if she says, "I couldn't do it without you; I couldn't live without you" I say, "Honey, I just couldn't live without you either. I just couldn't imagine being without you. I love you so much."

Gary Chapman: Rick, I would say that's a mutual expression of intimacy. That's relational intimacy happening. It might look different than intimacy looked when you were newlyweds and she didn't have this horrible disease.

Betsy: Like Rick mentioned, the kind of intimacy we had earlier in our marriages is gone. It's a different kind of intimacy and it may just be the way that we care for them, intervening on their behalf.

Compassion for a Spouse Who "Can't Do Anything"

Penny: Dennis will try to do something, maybe try his photography, or go to the computer or get the television so screwed up. And then he says, "I'm just Mr. Useless." And then you've got to deal with the heartache of knowing that we don't know what that feels like inside of them.

Sarah: Bob always comes back to, "I'm just so stupid. I'm not good for anybody" and he says that to me quite frequently. And I have to encourage him and tell him, "You're helpful."

Betsy: Brent built a log home for us from scratch. He was a great carpenter and rock layer and he'd never done any of that in his entire life. He hated to read, but he would read to learn how to do that. And so now he can't even hammer a nail. Sometimes he'll try to do something like that and that's when I get that glimpse of the sadness in him. Sometimes he'll just start crying. Like somebody was saying a minute ago, he feels useless. The hardest thing for me is when he does actually realize that he can't do anything.

Rick: Stephanie is always asking, "What can I do?" And the problem is that she gets so frustrated when she can't do it. She gets so agitated she gets nauseous. So, much of my life is trying to tell her, "Honey, please sit down and relax for a little bit." For someone like her who was so proactive and such a professional person and took such pride in her home, it's just absolutely devastating for her to find herself in this situation. Fortunately, she doesn't have a lot of times where she realizes exactly what's happened. She has periods of clarity, but they don't last too long. And she will just cry her eyes out whenever she thinks about what she's losing and what she's lost. It's the most difficult thing I've ever done in my 60-something years on this earth.

JoAnne: This is different from what a lot of you have mentioned, but Jerry doesn't seem to be aware of his situation, so he doesn't get frustrated. At least he doesn't express it to me if he's feeling frustrated or upset about anything.

Our takeaway: dementia patients who have preserved insight can get very frustrated by their inability to get things done, which in turn is heartrending for the care partner. This reminds us of a very important caregiving principle, especially when caring for a person with preserved insight: to the extent possible, realizing that it takes a lot of patience, do things with, not for, the person with dementia.

When insight is not preserved, as with Jerry (who has frontotemporal dementia), care partners can regard this as a blessing. Ed said, "Often I will ask Rebecca if she's happy, or if she's having a good day. Almost without fail, she'll say yes, often with an affirming nod of her head and a smile. In these moments I thank God that she has been spared the negative emotions that would accompany insight into her disease, like sadness, fear, and anger. At her present stage of the disease, she verbalizes a lot but it's impossible to understand 99 percent of what she says. If she remembered she was a speech pathologist, I think the inability to communicate would be very difficult for her to accept."

Humor

Sarah: Bob goes to adult daycare twice a week and one Friday he decided he needed to dress up. When we came home he said, "I need to change my clothes." He was gone for a long while. When he came out he said, "Does this look all right?" He was wearing a pair of my capri pants with his dress shoes and his black socks. And it was all I could do to contain myself. How he got my pants on I don't know. You have to laugh! There are some things that are just so funny, you have to laugh at them because they would never happen again in a lifetime.

JoAnne: Jerry has these little hallucinations. We have a person, Pete, who stays with him on the days that I babysit our little granddaughter. Jerry kept telling Pete that he was sure I was bringing home a Jeep. He was sitting in the front room looking out the window, waiting for me to bring home a Jeep. Pete normally brings him over to our son's house where I babysit late in the afternoon. But that day Jerry wouldn't leave the house. So Pete called me and said, "Jerry won't come over this afternoon, because he thinks you're coming home with either a Jeep or a red Corvette."

I don't have any idea where that came from, and I'm not going to be stopping at a dealership! He mentioned it again this morning. He said, "I think I hear my gift coming up the hill."

He's thinking a car is coming for him, so I hope Publishers Clearinghouse comes through!

WHAT HELPS YOU "KEEP ON KEEPING ON"?

Support Group

JoAnne: This support group has been a very good resource. I don't know if everybody has the opportunity to be a part of a group. You all have helped me.

Angela: It has been very helpful for me to be in this support group. My husband is still in the early stages and Penny said to me one time, "When you hear us talk about our spouses being further along and some of our trials, is that hard for you?" No, I find it very helpful to hear from all of you, so that when I get to that place, I have your words of wisdom. This support group has been very helpful to me in that way.

Betsy: Even though we're here in this group for ourselves, we're really doing this so we can be better care partners for them.

Sarah: A support group is absolutely wonderful. I don't know what I would do without this one.

Help from Others

Sarah: It's impossible to do it alone and I've learned not to be afraid to ask people for help. That was one of my hardest things because I was always a giver, doing for others. You have to accept that as a care partner you cannot do it alone. Ask for help if you need it.

Penny: So often people want to help, but they have no idea what to do. Thinking about what helps fill up my love tank is a good way to introduce that. I have plenty of people to come in to sweep the floors, but what I really need is to know that Dennis is okay and I can be off for a while. So it's important for me to tell somebody what I need.

Learning

Angela: I think knowledge is power. It has been very important to me to learn as much as I could about this disease.

Faith

Angela: My faith—I could not have gotten through the last two years without the peace that has come from my Savior.

Sarah: My strongest thing is my faith. I turn to God's Word every day because it gives me the strength as a caregiver to know that I'm not alone. That God is there and He's helping me.

Keeping the Promise

Betsy: The first thing that comes to my mind is my marriage vows to my husband. We said "for better or for worse" and this is obviously the worst. And we're to be loyal. We have to be there for them and they counted on it.

The Little Things

Troy: That little sentence that he gives you, or she gives you, that may not be a full sentence, but it means something—it's just sweet. So those little things, hold onto those and use them as motivation.

Choosing Hesed

Ed said to Rick, "You and Stephanie have been married 10 years, but you were in your mid-50s and she was in her mid-40s when you married. This is your second marriage and it was her first marriage. You've had fewer years of marriage than most of the people who are here. Has it been harder for you to hang in there? Do you think, given that this second marriage has turned out so differently, that you can hang in there with this?"

Rick: At first I thought about calling Stephanie's parents and telling them, "Your daughter is seriously ill. I cannot handle it. Can you come and get her?" I knew from what little relationship I had with them that they were too old, and I knew her brothers really didn't care, so she really didn't have anyone else.

She was not an easy person when we were first married, even before she became ill, but I think a lot of that was the beginning of her illness. It would have been very easy for me to say, "I just can't do it. The return on my emotional investment has been really poor."

> "I really feel our love has grown stronger because of this illness. She's become like a child to me, a child that I love, and someone I would do anything for." —RICK

But I really feel our love has grown stronger because of this illness. She's become like a child to me, a child that I love, and someone I would do anything for. Caregiving really has threatened my health. It has been an incredible sacrifice. I've had close family members who have passed away and I have not been able to go to their funerals, because she cannot travel anymore. A lot of sacrifices, but I just love her very, very much, love her as a wife, love

194

her in the childlike form that she finds herself. I'm so glad I never followed through on my initial thoughts of perhaps hanging it up.

Finding Meaning in Dementia Caregiving

Penny: I realized, not too long ago, that I was so glad that this was happening to Dennis instead of me, because I don't think he could bear this heartache. I just don't think he could do it, and I'm going to get through it somehow. I knew then that I loved him more than I had ever known, and I would never be able to say it, but I hoped he could feel it. I think we grow into this. I think it is the best part of ourselves. It really is the most important thing we'll ever do.

Sarah: God gives different people different gifts. You stop and think about it, isn't this the gift that He gave me, for caring? I can't imagine myself doing anything else in my life right now except taking care of Bob.

Troy: I see in every aspect that each of us has mentioned that we show our love by trying to support them, by advocating for them at the doctor's office, by making sure they are dressed properly before they leave. Like you said Sarah, we know if the shoe were on the other foot, they'd do it for us, and probably better.

Can I just share one quote from a book that I cherish? It's a quote from *Thoughtful Dementia Care: Understanding the Dementia Experience*: "A few carers said that they thought their spouse had dementia because they, the carers, were being punished by God. When dementia is in your family, it could be viewed instead as a divine gift to teach totally unselfish caring."[1] I think about that last sentence. We could look at it as we're being punished or we could turn it around and think of it as, this is our way to show unselfish love. I think that's what we all do.

Remember

Angela: I can still see the love in my husband's eyes and the love in his smile, for whatever small thing it might be. That smile will mean the world to me, so I want to really hold onto the memory of that as he progresses. We just hold on to whatever little thing it is that helps us to still have a part of them and who they were to us or are to us.

Troy: In the early stages they ask you something over and over and over again. Remember that, because one day down the road you will no longer hear their voice.

WRAPPING UP

Ed, speaking to Gary: One of the metaphors that stuck with me from *The 5 Love Languages®* book was the notion of an emotional love tank. When a married couple comes in for counseling, their emotional love tanks often have holes in them. I think the same metaphor applies to care partners, except maybe instead of a puncture it might be a gaping hole. Some of our group members have spoken very clearly of the emptiness of the tank and just how hard it is to keep it filled. I wonder if you might share your thoughts, given your many years of ex-

> "In the early stages they ask you something over and over and over again. Remember that, because one day down the road you will no longer hear their voice."
>
> —TROY

perience with this notion, and now that you've been with us in some support groups?

Gary: One of my thoughts is that all of us, no matter what our state in life, have the emotional need to feel loved by the most significant people in our lives. If you feel loved by the significant people in your life, the love tank is full, life is beautiful, and we can process things pretty well. If the love tank is empty, and you feel like nobody really cares, life can look pretty dark. I think much of the misbehavior of people often grows out of the fact that their love tank is empty. Their misbehavior is an effort to fill the love tank.

In your situation now, you're not receiving a whole lot of love response from the most significant person in your life, your spouse. But there are other significant people in your life—children or your parents might still be living or you have a close friend or two. I think a lot of people, particularly your close circle of friends, really do want to help, but they may not know how. I think there could be value in your sharing the concept of the love languages with the significant people in your life and saying, "Take the quiz and tell me what your love language is, and I'll take the quiz and tell you mine."

If they have information about what to do to make you feel loved, they are more likely to do that. If they knew, for example, that your love language was *Quality Time*, they may call you more often and say, "Can I take you to lunch or can I come over and chat with you for a while?" If you were to share the love languages concept with your circle of significant people, it might enhance everybody's relationships. Not just yours, but theirs as well.

The other point I make about the love languages in normal relationships is that we can receive love in all five languages; all of us can. You give heavy doses of the primary love language, then you sprinkle in the other four, kind of for extra credit. Whatever the stage of dementia, all five languages might be meaningful to a person. But if you can reflect on what their primary one might have been, that one might still be most meaningful to them, depending on what disease stage they're in.

The Journey No One Wants to Take

"When we are no longer able to change a situation,
we are challenged to change ourselves."
-VIKTOR FRANKL, *Man's Search for Meaning*

A NOTE FROM ED

"IT IS WHAT IT IS."

Those who have been with Rebecca on her journey with mild cognitive impairment and Alzheimer's disease recognize these words she would often say in response to questions such as, "How's your brain?" or "How are you doing?" I have often wondered what she would say about the last nine years of her life, what a journal might have reflected had she been able to keep one. She would not have asked, "Why me?" Rather she would have said, "Why not me?" just as she had when facing other trials in her life.

While some may say "why not me?" is an act of blind faith, for Rebecca, it would be an eyes-wide-open statement of trust in God. She would talk about being mad and sad. Rebecca has hated her Alzheimer's disease and has fought it every step of the way. She didn't like saying the "A word." It reminded her of who she wasn't, rather than who she was. As a person who preferred an orderly world, the progressive disorganization, even chaos, the disease caused was an immense frustration to her, especially early on. She would have been glad that a loss of insight accompanied the loss of function, and would have seen this as the merciful part of her disease. But more than mad, she would be sad, sad she couldn't grow old with me, sad she wouldn't see all her daughters grow up and realize their potential. She would have been sad that she couldn't see her grandchildren do the same.

Rebecca cherished children. Holding a crying baby, her own or those of others in the church nursery, walking and rocking them whispering a gentle "sh-sh-sh" till they fell asleep in her arms, is what she loved to do, perhaps more than anything else in the world. She would echo a word of thanks that she was able to touch the lives of her grandsons, Paul and Isaiah. They certainly have touched hers.

Perhaps more than anything else, Rebecca would express gratitude for the love and compassionate care she has received from her family, friends, and caregivers, that she hasn't been a burden but rather the recipient of *hesed*, the intentional, sacrificial love from those whose lives she touched with her gentle spirit, and in return have served her with a sad joyfulness. She would also be humbled that her journey with Alzheimer's disease would touch so many lives, would be an encouragement to other people diagnosed with dementia, bearing witness that one's life can have meaning, that there is much to be given, even in the face of an incurable neurodegenerative disease.

Like Rebecca, I have also learned to trust God. The best way I can explain this is with a driving metaphor. A car has both a windshield to look through when driving ahead, and a rearview mirror to show what is behind. When I look into the rearview mirror and see the life I've shared with Rebecca, from the sweetness of our relationship, to the joy of our children and now grandchildren, my response is one of gratitude, recognizing that the good things in life are indeed a blessing from God.

Looking through the windshield at what's ahead, I see a road that has twists and turns, darkness, and uncertainty. It is the journey down the path not chosen. My heart tells me that the God I praise looking in the rearview mirror is a good God, whereas I question the character and power of the God that is ahead. My head says there cannot be two Gods, a good one and a bad one, they must be one and the same. It is out of this struggle that my faith has been strengthened; and trust, the noun, has given rise to trust, the verb. And like Rebecca, I have seen good come from this journey of hers with Alzheimer's disease. My daughters, Erin, Leah, Carrie, and I are closer than ever. We have learned to hold one another up. We depend on one another. Other relationships have also been strengthened with family members, friends, and coworkers. Their love has been poured out willingly and freely.

The Memory Counseling Program, now a program of Wake Forest Baptist Health, did not exist five years ago, and would not exist had Rebecca not developed Alzheimer's disease. This counseling program has now served hundreds of individuals, couples, and families impacted by dementia through counseling sessions and support groups. This book, and the five love languages, we (Debbie, Gary, and I) hope, will be a valuable resource for those who find themselves in what often feels like a dark, lonely place, whether it be the person with dementia, or their care partner, or someone trying to understand how to help. And finally, we hope you, the reader, will find *shalom*, the Hebrew word for peace, through these words that have been shaped by the experiences of those on the dementia journey.

A NOTE FROM DEBBIE

I did not expect the experience of writing this book to change me, but it did. I have been deeply touched by the sincere and self-less love of the incredible care partners I have come to admire so much. Their loyal love, their tears, their gut-level honesty about their struggles, and their good humor in spite of it all showed me, by comparison, how poorly I love. The example of these care partners challenges me to do a better job of loving my family, friends, and everyone who crosses my path, especially those who are most difficult to love: those with no desire or ability to love me back. As a person with a deep faith in God, I've long known the importance of loving others, but these care partners now inspire and motivate me to take love to a new level. Gracie's story in particular showed me that when love is truly given from the heart, even when that love is spurned or goes unreciprocated, the giver can still find fulfillment and sometimes even joy. She is living proof that we all need to both receive *and* give love.

Many care partners say that there is nothing extraordinary about their sacrificial love and loyal care of their loved one. They say they are just doing what they know their loved one would have done for them if the tables were turned. Selflessness is now a way of life for them. Most of them did not start out with this mindset, however. For many, it began as a journey of tears and fears and moments of despair, powered by courage and the sheer willpower to keep stepping forward into the unknown. They didn't bail out; they chose to stay, and they continue to stay, out of love and loyalty.

Just as a muscle grows a tiny bit stronger each time a weight is lifted, I have come to believe that as care partners choose to do the hard thing, to intentionally love, over and over, though it may be imperceptible to them, they are slowly changed in positive ways. Certainly, every care partner I know has good days and not-so-good days as they continue in the daily grind of caregiving; not one of them does this perfectly and none would say that he or she has "arrived." Yet, those who have journeyed long as care partners are not the people they once were. Because of the disease that invaded their lives and rerouted everything, they are, paradoxically, *better* now than before—stronger, more confident, more patient, and more resilient. But not one of them chose this path. No one would ever choose it; dementia is truly a journey no one wants to take.

As a health educator and health promoter, I also think about the dementia journey in its wider context, the Alzheimer's epidemic that is ramping up all around us. Currently 5.4 million Americans have AD.[1] Because advancing age is the biggest risk factor, now that the baby boomers are becoming senior adults and people are living longer than ever before, the number of people with AD is only expected to climb. If a cure is not found by 2050, it is estimated that by then at least 13.8 million Americans will have the disease, with other estimates as high as 16 million.[1] If these predictions come to pass, the cost of AD and other dementias, currently $236 billion annually, will skyrocket as well. Projections for 2050 place costs at more than $1 trillion.[1] How will our nation respond to this tsunami of dementia patients?

If readers carry away just one message from this book, I hope it is, in the words of the researcher in chapter 4, that "the emotional life of an Alzheimer's patient is alive and well." I hope too, that we have shown that this is true even when a person's demeanor would lead us to a different conclusion. In light of this, it is incredibly sad that, according to the studies cited in chapter 3, about half of all dementia patients are abused or mistreated. Clearly, far too few care partners are as selfless, loving, and inspiring as the ones we encountered during the writing of this book. The disturbing question that must be asked is, if the number of patients triples by 2050 as predicted, how safely will they fare? Will widespread knowledge of their emotional awareness be enough to ensure that they will be treated kindly and in ways that preserve their dignity? Or will exorbitant costs and the sheer volume of patients so burden the healthcare system and weary society as a whole that persons with dementia will be devalued and their welfare jeopardized?

Throughout the chapters of this book, the word *hesed* has been a recurring theme. We have used this word to describe the "gold standard" of dementia care—the loyal, merciful, intentional love that intervenes on behalf of loved ones and comes to their rescue. In antiquity, this Hebrew word was used to describe the love of God Himself for humanity. There has never been a higher love than the *hesed* of God, and it is His love, many care partners tell us, that empowers them to love the person in their care so well.

Unless a cure is found, it is certain that dementia will continue to unravel one family tapestry after another in the years ahead. As a nation and as communities, we must begin now to think proactively about how we will compassionately protect, legislate for, and advocate for the millions on the dementia journey. If we accept nothing short of *hesed* as our guiding principle, and if we collectively will it so, ageism, mistreatment, and abuse will find no place in the epidemic that lies ahead.

I can think of no greater legacy for this book than to help create this kind of future for all those on the dementia journey.

40 Ways to Say "I Love You" in Middle- and Late-Stage Dementia

Research by Logsdon and Teri[1] suggests that there are 20 "pleasant activities" that people with dementia enjoy. We have combined these activities with a list from *Creating Moments of Joy*[2] by Jolene Brackey, and added some of our own ideas. Below, we have grouped all of these suggestions within the framework of the five love languages. As you have opportunity, let the list guide you in creatively expressing love. Remember that the further along a person is in their disease, the simpler your expressions of love must be.

ACTS OF KINDNESS (ACTS OF SERVICE)

☐ Look them in the eye when they speak to you no matter what they say or how they say it.

☐ Include them in conversations (rather than talk about them as if they are not present).

☐ Let them help in the kitchen, around the house, wherever and whenever they want to contribute.

☐ Help them groom (makeup, shave, comb hair, pick out clothing).

☐ Advocate for them.

☐ Smile at them as you come and go.

☐ People with AD have trouble making decisions, yet feel devalued if not allowed to participate in decisions that affect them. So, let them choose between two options you have pre-approved (red shirt/blue shirt).

☐ When they complain or are delusional, empathize ("I am so sorry that happened"), then gently distract them with something pleasant.

☐ Let them be right.

WORDS OF AFFIRMATION

☐ Tell them, "I love you."

☐ Answer each repeated question as if it were being asked for the first time.

☐ Talk to them (even if they can't talk back)—about their life growing up, marriage, children, grandchildren, work, and hobbies.

☐ Tell them they look handsome/beautiful (even if it's the same outfit they wore yesterday and it's dirty).

☐ Help them write a card or letter and sign it.

☐ Sing them to sleep.

☐ Tell them that you have taken care of everything.

☐ Tell them you are proud of all the things they accomplished in life.

☐ Brag about them to others while they are present.

RECEIVING GIFTS

☐ Give them a piece of chocolate, ice cream cone, chocolate chip cookie, or whatever they love.

☐ Give them a surprise package to open.

☐ Send a card to them in the mail.

☐ Give them an iPod loaded with music from their teen and young adult years.

☐ Bring them a coloring book with some markers or crayons.

☐ Be generous with the gift of your time.

QUALITY MOMENTS (QUALITY TIME)

☐ Read to them or, if they can, have them read to you or a grandchild.

☐ Reminisce about old times and important events of history as you look at a photo album or family movies.

☐ Watch a favorite movie over and over.

☐ Go for a ride in the car.

☐ Bake some cookies.

☐ Laugh and giggle—they may join in.

☐ Color in a coloring book or do a puzzle with them.

☐ Tell stories.

PHYSICAL TOUCH

☐ Hold hands and take a walk.

☐ Give a hug (and kiss, if appropriate).

☐ Sit close by or hold them if they're afraid, angry, or agitated.

☐ Rub their feet or their back or gently stroke their cheek.

☐ Let them hold a baby, puppy, or doll.

☐ File and/or put polish on their fingernails and toenails.

☐ Dance or move to music with them.

☐ Massage their hands and arms with lotion.

Appendix B

For Those Who Want to Know More

Lobes of the Brain (chapter 4)
Attachment (chapter 5)
Non-Alzheimer's Dementias (chapter 6)

LOBES OF THE BRAIN[1,2]

The brain is highly complex. As mentioned in chapter 4, no brain area ever works in isolation. Keep this in mind as you consider the specific functions of each lobe of the brain noted below. Each lobe is a vital component of the brain's intricate network of interconnected neurons (nerve cells).

The Frontal Lobes: The Management Center

The frontal lobes comprise the management center of the brain. These lobes govern the brain functions that characterize the different aspects of the human personality, including:

- Impulse control
- Social behavior (much of which is based on our morals and values)
- Motivation
- Reasoning

- Judgment
- Insight
- Executive function

Executive function includes the ability to pay attention, concentrate, stay on task, plan, problem solve, and multitask. "Executive functions are the most . . . complex of biological functions in the known universe," wrote Dr. J. Riley McCarten. "Almost half of the brain—the frontal lobes—is dedicated to executive functions."[3] The frontal lobes are also involved in language expression, the control of movement, smell, appetite, and taste. These lobes also house the mirror neurons. "Mirror neurons," Dr. Christina Hugenschmidt explained, "are what make you feel sad when somebody else is crying. They enable you to take someone else's perspective—to have empathy. Empathy means I can notice something and say, 'That's what she would want,' which means that you're able to think about it from someone else's perspective."

Damage to different parts of the frontal lobes results in various problems. When Broca's area, in the left frontal lobe, is damaged, a person has difficulty with verbal expression. If the middle part of the frontal lobe is damaged, people become apathetic and unmotivated, which may seem like depression, but is not. If the front part is damaged, disinhibition occurs, making the person prone to argue, swear, or do socially inappropriate things, without the insight to understand that what they've said or done is embarrassing or unfitting.

The Temporal Lobes: The Memory and Emotion Center

The temporal lobes occupy the lower half of the brain, beneath the temples extending back towards the ears on both sides of the head. These lobes are important for memory, for integrating hearing and speech, and for understanding language. A hippocampus

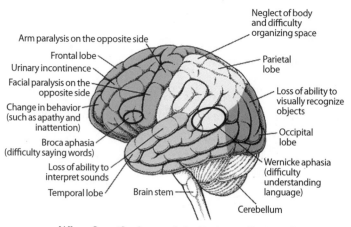

Arm paralysis on the opposite side

Frontal lobe

Urinary incontinence

Facial paralysis on the opposite side

Change in behavior (such as apathy and inattention)

Broca aphasia (difficulty saying words)

Loss of ability to interpret sounds

Temporal lobe

Brain stem

Neglect of body and difficulty organizing space

Parietal lobe

Loss of ability to visually recognize objects

Occipital lobe

Wernicke aphasia (difficulty understanding language)

Cerebellum

When Specific Areas of the Brain are Damaged

From the Merck Manual Consumer Version (known as the Merck Manual in the US and Canada and the MSD Manual in the rest of the world), edited by Robert Porter. Copyright 2015 by Merck Sharp & Dohme Corp., a subsidiary of Merck & Co., Inc, Kenilworth, NJ. Available at http://www.merckmanuals.com/consumer. Accessed February 3, 2016.

is housed in each temporal lobe. The hippocampi are important for forming and storing new memories and for retrieving long-term memories, thus they help us learn new information. The hippocampi also process verbal memories (words that are read, spoken, or heard), and visual memories (objects, faces, and places). The most classic symptom of Alzheimer's disease, memory loss, is caused by damage to the hippocampi. Near each hippocampus, both temporal lobes house another structure called the amygdala, which integrates emotions, emotional learning, and emotional memory. (Many of our memories have an emotional component, hence the term *emotional memory*.) The amygdalae, which govern all human emotion, also enable us to recognize the emotions we see in facial expressions. The temporal lobes allow us to be aware of music and to link music to emotionally important people and life events. Due to damage in the temporal lobes, individuals with Alzheimer's may forget the people closest to them and lose the emotional memories associated with loving and caring about those people.

The Parietal Lobes: The Internal "GPS"

The parietal lobes comprise the upper half of the brain toward the back. They are located behind the frontal and above the temporal lobes. These lobes interpret information from our five senses and aspects of visual perception that tell us about size, shape, color, and depth of objects. The parietal lobes also assist in recognition of familiar objects and faces. Someone with dementia that involves the parietal lobes might walk up to a stranger and talk to them as if he or she were a friend from the past. The stranger likely had a similar face shape as someone known in the past, but with parietal lobe damage, the PWD no longer remembered the precise details of what that person looked like.

Along with the temporal lobes, the parietal lobes enable mathematical skills and language comprehension. The parietal lobes also assist with visual-spatial function. This function enables us to orient ourselves in three-dimensional space, including telling right from left, which is important in all physical activity, including everyday activities such as going up and down stairs and driving. Impaired visual-spatial function is one reason individuals with AD eventually have difficulty with driving, a complex activity that involves the integration of visual-spatial, memory, and language functions. Making a judgment about a patient's driving ability is one of the most challenging assessments a dementia doctor has to make, and losing the ability to drive is one of the hardest parts of the AD journey.

The Occipital Lobes: The Computers that Process Vision

The occipital lobes are located at the very back of the brain and are responsible for the processing of the visual information seen by the eyes. The occipital lobes are not usually affected in Alzheimer's disease but they do play a role in a rare type of dementia called posterior cortical atrophy (PCA). PCA often begins with difficulties with visual tasks such as reading. Experts have not yet determined whether PCA is a unique type of dementia or a variation of Alzheimer's disease.[4]

ATTACHMENT

Over the last decade, a great deal of progress has been made in understanding the brain basis of relationships, also referred to as "interpersonal neurobiology." The work of Dr. Bonnie Badenoch, a marriage and family therapist and instructor at Portland State University, has been foundational in this understanding.[5,6] She describes several components that help form and maintain our attachments to our loved ones. Attachment, simply defined, is the emotional bond between people. Attachments begin at birth—in fact, early attachments are the most important—and are formed throughout childhood, adolescence, and adulthood.

In the beginning of chapter 5, we talked about dopamine, the brain chemical that naturally rewards us when we give or receive love. Dr. Badenoch says dopamine is not only involved in reward, but also in seeking relationship with the people in our lives with whom we need connection. She calls this "the seeking system." As noted in chapter 5, when we're disconnected from those we love, we experience separation distress, panic, and grief. We naturally seek reconnection, and the harder it is to reconnect, the more the seeker will emotionally and physically cling to those with whom he or she is trying to connect. In the absence of reconnection, the seeker will express negative emotions such as anger (even rage), sadness, and anxiety. This may be the very underlying reason for many of the negative behaviors, including agitation and the desire to "go home," that we often see in those with dementia. Often, family members respond to this emotional and physical clinginess by pushing away, when what's really needed is attachment and connection.

In the context of persons with dementia, as memory fades, dementia progressively disconnects the affected individual from their core attachments with parents, siblings, spouse/partner, and children. In turn, loved ones are experiencing similar attachment losses with their spouse or parent in a process of ongoing grief. Many of the challenging thoughts, emotions, and behaviors seen in the person with Alzheimer's and their family are the result of attachment loss.

The five love languages are tools that help loved ones reestablish or maintain as much connection as possible, always mindful that Alzheimer's is a neurodegenerative disease. This means, using the tapestry metaphor, that the disease never stops its relentless unraveling of the attachment "fibers" that are so vital to our identity as mother, father, brother, sister, husband, wife, son, daughter, and friend.

NON-ALZHEIMER'S DEMENTIAS

Dementia is an umbrella term that encompasses a wide range of symptoms associated with cognitive decline, including memory loss, the inability to complete complex tasks, and changes in personality, mood, and behavior. There are many types of dementia. Alzheimer's disease, as readers now know, is the most common dementia. Other types of dementia include the following:

Frontotemporal dementia (FTD) is an umbrella term for conditions that cause portions of the frontal and temporal lobes of the brain to shrink and lose function. FTD is the fourth most common type of dementia and typically affects younger people. FTD affects more men than women, with people generally living an average of 6-7 years after diagnosis. It can occur along with other types of dementia or neurodegenerative diseases such as Parkinson's disease and ALS (Lou Gehrig's disease). Because symptoms mimic other conditions, FTD is sometimes misdiagnosed as Alzheimer's disease, Parkinson's disease, manic-depression, obsessive-compulsive disorder, or schizophrenia. The most common FTD disorders affect behavior and/or language.

Lewy body dementia (LBD) is an umbrella term for forms of dementia that result from the presence of Lewy bodies in the brain. Lewy bodies are abnormal deposits of protein. LBD typically begins after age 50 with the lifespan after diagnosis averaging five to eight years, but ranging from 2–20 years, depending on the stage of the disease at diagnosis. Although LBD is the third most common dementia, it is often unrecognized and can be misdiagnosed because, depending on when symptoms appear, it may resemble a psychotic disorder like schizophrenia, Alzheimer's disease, or Parkinson's disease. For some people, the first symptoms may be hallucinations, paranoid delusions, and REM sleep disorder. Patients also experience unpredictable ups and downs in attention, concentration, alertness, wakefulness, and cognitive function.

Others initially have difficulty with executive function (planning, problem solving, multitasking, and judgment) and visual-spatial problems that resemble Alzheimer's disease. Other symptoms common in Alzheimer's, such as memory loss, language difficulties, apathy, and anxiety often occur, but may not be problematic until late in the disease, if at all. For still others, LBD begins with Parkinson's disease–like symptoms that affect both movement and body function. Cognitive symptoms occur later.

Mixed dementia means having more than one type of dementia simultaneously. About half of those with Alzheimer's disease have evidence of another type of dementia. Recent studies suggest that mixed dementia is more common than previously thought. [7]

Parkinson's disease dementia (PDD) occurs in 50–80 percent of those with Parkinson's disease. As with Lewy body dementia, PDD results from abnormal deposits of protein known as Lewy bodies. PDD symptoms can include irritability and anxiety, sleep problems, changes in concentration, judgment, and memory, as well as depression, delusions, and visual hallucinations.

Reversible dementias illumine the importance of seeking an early medical evaluation when memory loss or other cognitive problems occur. When caused by disease or injury, dementia is irreversible. Some other kinds of dementia, however, can be treated medically and reversed. According to the Alzheimer's Association, one review of many studies found that 9 percent of people with dementia-like symptoms actually did not have dementia, but potentially reversible conditions. The most common cause of reversible memory loss is depression. Other causes of potentially reversible memory and cognitive symptoms include drugs (prescription medications or illicit drugs), alcohol, underactive thyroid gland, normal pressure hydrocephalus, brain tumor, and vitamin B12 deficiency.

Vascular dementia is the second most common type of dementia, accounting for up to 20 percent of cases. It results from reduced blood flow to the brain, often after multiple strokes. Vascular dementia coexists with another type of dementia in about 50 percent of cases (see *Mixed Dementia*). Unlike the dementias described above, which slowly progress over a period of years, vascular dementia often has an abrupt onset following a stroke. However, if an individual experiences a series of "mini-strokes" over a period of months to years, vascular dementia can progress slowly. Recent research has revealed that vascular dementia can also result from small vessel disease. Small vessel disease results from damage sustained by the small blood vessels deep in the brain, most often due to high blood pressure.

The cognitive functions affected by vascular dementia are similar to those impaired by AD but depend on the location of the stroke. For instance, while memory loss is seen in all cases of AD, it may or may not be present with vascular dementia.

Appendix C

Suggested Resources

THE 5 LOVE LANGUAGES®

Books, eBooks, audiobooks, DVDs, and mobile apps
available at www.5lovelanguages.com

The 5 Love Languages:® The Secret to Love That Lasts, Gary Chapman, Northfield Publishing, Chicago, 2015.

The 5 Love Languages,® Singles Edition, Gary D. Chapman, Northfield Publishing, Chicago, 2014.

Online Love Languages Quiz: http://www.5lovelanguages.com/profile/

ALZHEIMER'S DISEASE

Reference Books

The 36-Hour Day: A Family Guide to Caring for People Who Have Alzheimer's Disease, Related Dementias, and Memory Loss. Nancy L. Mace, MA and Peter V. Rabins, MD, MPH, Grand Central Life & Style; 5th edition, September 25, 2012.

Mayo Clinic Guide to Alzheimer's Disease: The Essential Resource for Treatment, Coping and Caregiving. Petersen, R., ed., Rochester, MN: Mayo Clinic Health Solutions, 2009.

The Alzheimer's Action Plan. P. Murali Doraiswamy, MD, Lisa P. Gwyther, MSW, and Tina Adler, St. Martin's Press, New York, NY, 1st edition, April 2008.

Books for Care Partners and Persons with Dementia

Living with Alzheimer's & Other Dementias: 101 Stories of Caregiving, Coping, and Compassion. Amy Newmark and Angela Timashenka Geiger, 1st Edition, Chicken Soup for the Soul Publishing, Ltd., Cos Cob, CT, 2014.

Coping with Behavior Change in Dementia: A Family Caregiver's Guide. Beth Spencer and Laurie White, 1st Edition, April 3, 2015.

Creating Moments of Joy for the Person with Alzheimer's or Dementia: A Journal for Caregivers, Jolene Brackey, 4th Edition, Purdue University Press, West Lafayette, IN, 2007.

Healing Your Grieving Heart When Someone You Care About Has Alzheimer's: 100 Practical Ideas for Families, Friends, and Caregivers, Alan D. Wolfelt PhD and Kirby J. Duvall MD, Companion Press, Ft. Collins, CO, 2014.

Living Your Best with Early-Stage Alzheimer's: An Essential Guide, Lisa Snyder MSW LCSW, Sunrise River Press, North Branch, MN, 2010.

Practical Dementia Care, Peter V. Rabins, Constantine G. Lykestos, and Cynthia D. Steele (ed), 3rd edition, Oxford University Press, April 29, 2016.

Thoughtful Dementia Care: Understanding the Dementia Experience, Jennifer Ghent-Fuller, 1st Edition, Thoughtful Dementia Care, Inc., 2012.

When Caring Takes Courage: A Compassionate, Interactive Guide for Alzheimer's and Dementia Caregivers, Mara Botonis, Outskirts Press, Inc., 2014.

Books for Children

What's Happening to Grandpa? Maria Shriver, Little, Brown Books for Young Readers, 2004.

Always My Grandpa: A Story for Children about Alzheimer's Disease, Linda Scacco, Magination Press, 2005.

Wilfrid Gordon McDonald Partridge, Mem Fox, Kane/Miller Book Publishers, 1989.

Resources from the National Institute on Aging

Alzheimer's Disease: Unraveling the Mystery, National Institute on Aging, Publication No. 08-3782. Download PDF at https://www.nia.nih.gov/alzheimers/publication/alzheimers-disease-unraveling-mystery/more-information.

Caring for a Person with Alzheimer's Disease: Your Easy-to-Use Guide from the National Institute on Aging, Publication Number 09-6173, March 2010. Order hard copy or download PDF from Contact Alzheimer's Disease Education and Referral (ADEAR) Center 1-800-438-4380. www.nia.nih.gov/alzheimers.

Available online or as PDF download from https://www.nia.nih.gov/alzheimers

Alzheimer's Disease Fact Sheet

Alzheimer's Disease Genetics Fact Sheet

Alzheimer's Disease Medications Fact Sheet

Forgetfulness: Knowing When to Ask for Help

Legal and Financial Planning for People with Alzheimer's Disease Fact Sheet

Understanding Memory Loss: What to Do When You Have Trouble Remembering

Websites

Alzheimer's Association. http://www.alz.org

Alzheimer's Disease Education and Referral Center (ADEAR). https://www.nia.nih.gov/alzheimers/

Alzheimer's Foundation of America. http://www.alzfdn.org

AARP Home & Family Caregiving. http://www.aarp.org/home-family/caregiving/

The Family Caregiver Alliance. https://www.caregiver.org

The Hartford Publications Home and Car Safety Guides
https://www.thehartford.com/resources/mature-market-excellence/
publications-on-aging

Alzheimer's Caregiver Page
https://www.nlm.nih.gov/medlineplus/alzheimerscaregivers.html

Guidelines for initiating meaningful, quality home visits with people who
have Alzheimer's disease and related dementia. http://www.wistatedocu
ments.org/cdm/ref/collection/p267601coll4/id/157

Alzheimer's Association Resource Listing: http://www.alz.org/library/lists
.asp#useful

Alzheimer's Disease International: http://www.alz.co.uk/

Videos, Movies, and Documentaries

Accepting the Challenge: Providing the Best Care for People with Dementia
(produced by Alzheimer's North Carolina, Inc.). http://www.healthpro
press.com/product/accepting-the-challenge/

Inside the Brain: Unraveling the Mystery of Alzheimer's Disease. https://www.
nia.nih.gov/alzheimers/alzheimers-disease-video

*About Dementia Videos (Dementia 101, Teepa's GEMS, Brain Changes,
Challenging Behaviors, Meaningful Activities, Music).* Teepa Snow—Positive Approach to Brain Change. http://teepasnow.com/resources/tee-
pa-tips-videos/

The Forgetting—A Portrait of Alzheimer's. http://www.pbs.org/theforget-
ting/watch/

Alive Inside (Henry's Story). YouTube.com

The Alzheimer's Project, HBO Documentary. HBO.com/alzheimers/

I'll Be Me (the Glen Campbell Sunset Tour). http://glencampbellmovie
.com

Still Alice Trailer. http://sonyclassics.com/stillalice/

Newsletters

Caregiver, newsletter of the Duke Alzheimer's Family Support Program. Written by Lisa Gwyther, LCSW and Bobbi Matchar, MSW, available at: http://www.dukefamilysupport.org/

Perspectives, quarterly newsletter for people with dementia and their care partners. Written by Lisa Snyder, LCSW, UCSD Shiley-Marcos Alzheimer's Disease Research Center, available by request from: lsnyder@ucsd.edu

OTHER DEMENTIAS

Frontotemporal Dementia

Books and Booklets

What If It's Not Alzheimer's? A Caregiver's Guide to Dementia, Gary Radin and Lisa Radin, Prometheus Books, 3rd edition, 2014.

Frontotemporal Disorders: Information for Patients, Families, and Caregivers, National Institute of Neurological Disorders and Stroke, Publication No. 14-6361. Download PDF or order hard copy at https://www.nia.nih.gov/alzheimers/publication/frontotemporal-disorders/basics-frontotemporal-disorders

Websites

The Association for Frontotemporal Degeneration (AFTD). http://www.theaftd.org

FTD Care Partnering. ttp://ftdsupport.com

UCSF Medical Center. http://memory.ucsf.edu/ftd/

FTD Resource Page. https://www.nia.nih.gov/alzheimers/publication/frontotemporal-disorders-resource-list

Lewy Body Dementia

Books & Booklets

A Caregiver's Guide to Lewy Body Dementia, Helen Buell Whitworth and James Whitworth, Demos Health, 2010.

Lewy Body Dementia: Information for Patients, Families, and Professionals, National Institute of Neurological Disorders and Stroke, Publication No. 15-7907. Download PDF or order hard copy at https://www.nia.nih.gov/alzheimers/publication/lewy-body-dementia/introduction

Websites and Other

Lewy Body Dementia Association. www.lewybodydementia.org/

NINDS Dementia With Lewy Bodies Page
http://www.ninds.nih.gov/disorders/dementiawithlewybodies/dementiawithlewybodies.htm

Lewy Body Dementia, Mayo Clinic website, http://www.mayoclinic.org/diseases-conditions/lewy-body-dementia/basics/definition/CON-20025038?p=1

Lewy Body Digest e-newsletter. Subscribe at https://www.lbda.org/content/sign-lewy-body-digest-0

Vascular Dementia

National Stroke Association: http://www.stroke.org/we-can-help/survivors/stroke-recovery/post-stroke-conditions/cognition/vascular-dementia

National Institute of Neurological Disorders and Stroke: http://www.ninds.nih.gov/disorders/multi_infarct_dementia/multi_infarct_dementia.htm

Notes

Chapter 1: Ed and Rebecca: A Love Story

1. Alzheimer's Association, "Younger/Early Onset Alzheimer's," http://www.alz.org.
2. George Kraus, *Helping the Alzheimer's Patient: Plain Talk and Practical Tools* (DVD), presented through PESI, copyright 2011, MEDS PDN, Eau Claire, WI.
3. Alzheimer's Association, "2016 Alzheimer's Disease Facts and Figures," http://www.alz.org/documents_custom/2016-facts-and-figures.pdf, 10, 17, 18, 19, 30, 32.

Chapter 2: Love: It's All in Your Head

1. Gary Chapman, *The 5 Love Languages®: The Secret to Love that Lasts* (Chicago: Northfield Publishing, 2015), 31–32.
2. *Strong's Exhaustive Concordance of the Bible*, "Hesed." Strong's number 2617.
3. Lois Tverberg, "Hesed: Enduring, Eternal, Undeserved Love," Our Rabbi Jesus (blog), May 2, 2012, http://ourrabbijesus.com/hesed-enduring-eternal-undeserved-love/.
4. Chapman, *The 5 Love Languages®*, 35–115.
5. "Dementia and the Brain," Alzheimer's Society, Factsheet 456LP, last reviewed September 2014, https://www.alzheimers.org.uk/site/scripts/documents_info .php?documentID=114.
6. S.J. Cutler. "Worries about getting Alzheimer's: who's concerned?", *Am J Alzheimers Dis Other Demen* 30, no. 6 (2015): 591–8. doi: 10.1177/1533317514568889. Epub 2015 Feb 4.
7. Maia Szalavitz, "Friends With Benefits: Being Highly Social Cuts Dementia Risk by 70%," *Time*, May 2, 2011, http://healthland.time.com/2011/05/02/ friends-with-benefits-being-highly-social-cuts-dementia-risk-by-70/.
8. Honor Whiteman, "Alzheimer's Association International Conference 2015: the highlights," *Medical News Today*, July 23, 2015, http://www.medicalnews today.com/articles/297228.php.
9. Tjalling Jan Holwerda et al., "Feelings of loneliness, but not social isolation, predict dementia onset: results from the Amsterdam Study of the Elderly (AMSTEL)," *J Neurol Neurosurg Psychiatry* 85, no. 2 (2014): 135–42.

10. Thai Nguyen, "Hacking Into Your Happy Chemicals: Dopamine, Serotonin, Endorphins and Oxytocin," *Huffington Post*, http://www.huffingtonpost.com/thai-nguyen/hacking-into-your-happy-c_b_6007660.html/. Updated: December 20, 2014.

11. Chapman, *The 5 Love Languages*®, 156.

12. James Beauregard, "Dementia: Behavioral Health Assessments and Interventions for Practitioners," Cross Country Education Seminar, October 9, 2015, Greensboro, NC. Workbook, 94.

13. Gary W. Small et al., "Diagnosis and treatment of Alzheimer disease and related disorders: consensus statement of the American Association for Geriatric Psychiatry, the Alzheimer's Association, and the American Geriatrics Society," *JAMA* 278, no. 16 (1997): 4–6.

Chapter 3: Alzheimer's Disease Puts Love to the Test

1. George Kraus, *Helping the Alzheimer's Patient: Plain Talk and Practical Tools* (DVD), presented through PESI, copyright 2011, MEDS PDN, Eau Claire, WI.

2. Nancy L. Mace and Peter V. Rabins, *The 36-Hour Day: A Family Guide for People Who Have Alzheimer's Disease, Related Dementias, and Memory Loss* (Baltimore: The Johns Hopkins University Press, 2011), 37.

3. Kraus, *Helping the Alzheimer's Patient: Plain Talk and Practical Tools*.

4. Carole B. Larken, "Me and My Alzheimer's Shadow," http://www.alzheimersreadingroom.com.

5. Peter V. Rabins, foreword to *The Longest Loss: Alzheimer's Disease and Dementia*, eds. Kenneth J. Doka and Amy S. Tucci (Washington, D.C.: Hospice Foundation of America, 2015), iii–iv.

6. Alzheimer's Association, "2016 Alzheimer's Disease Facts and Figures," http://www.alz.org/documents_custom/2016-facts-and-figures.pdf, 32.

7. Alzheimer's Association, "2016 Alzheimer's Disease Facts and Figures," 36.

8. U.S. Department on Health and Human Services, Office of Women's Health, "Caregiver Stress: Frequently Asked Questions," www.womenshealth.gov.

9. Alzheimer's Association, "2016 Alzheimer's Disease Facts and Figures," 36.

10. C. Cooper, A. Selwood, M. Blanchard, Z. Walker, R. Blizard, and G. Livingston. (2009). "Abuse of people with dementia by family carers: representative cross sectional survey," *British Medical Journal, 338*, b155.

11. A. Wiglesworth, L. Mosqueda, R. Mulnard, S.Liao, L. Gibbs, and W. Fitzgerald, "Screening for abuse and neglect of people with dementia," *Journal of the American Geriatrics Society* 58, no. 3 (2010): 493–500.

12. Johns Hopkins Medicine, "Spouses Who Care For Partners With Dementia at Sixfold Higher Risk of Same Fate: Stress of caregiving may be to blame," press release May 5, 2010, http://www.hopkinsmedicine.org.

13. Richard Schulz and Scott R. Beach, "Caregiving as a Risk Factor for Mortality: The Caregiver Health Effects Study," *JAMA* 282, no. 23 (1999): 2215–2219.

14. Alzheimer's Association, "2015 Alzheimer's Disease Facts and Figures," 39.

15. National Institute on Aging, National Institutes of Health, *Alzheimer's Disease: Unraveling the Mystery*. Publication No. 08-3782. https://www.nia.nih.gov/alzheimers/publication.

16. Alan D Wolfelt, "Dispelling Five Common Myths About Grief" (seminar handout), Exploring Complicated Mourning: Sudden Death and Trauma Loss, seminar presented at Hospice of Davidson County, Lexington, NC, October 21, 2015.

17. Pauline Boss, *Loving Someone Who Has Dementia: How to Find Hope While Coping with Stress and Grief* (San Francisco: Jossey-Bass, 2011), 165.

18. Chapman, *The 5 Love Languages®: The Secret to Love that Lasts* (Chicago: Northfield Publishing, 2010), 44.

19. Ibid., 53.

20. Ibid., 78.

21. Ibid., 170.

22. Alzheimer's Association, "2016 Alzheimer's Disease Facts and Figures," 19.

23. Alzheimer's Association, "Cultural Competence," http://www.alz.org/Resources/Diversity/downloads/GEN_EDU-10steps.pdf.

24. Mace and Rabins, *The 36-Hour Day*, 407.

25. Debbie Barr, *A Season at Home: The Joy of Fully Sharing Your Child's Critical Years* (Grand Rapids: Zondervan, 1993), 168.

26. Lauren G. Collins and Kristine Swartz, "Caregiver Care," *American Family Physician* 83, no. 11 (2011): 1310. www.aafp.org/afp.

27. Johns Hopkins Medicine, "Spouses Who Care For Partners With Dementia at Sixfold Higher Risk of Same Fate: Stress of caregiving may be to blame," press release May 5, 2010, http://www.hopkinsmedicine.org.

28. Akemi Hirano et al., "Influence of regular exercise on subjective sense of burden and physical symptoms in community-dwelling caregivers of dementia patients: A randomized controlled trial," *Arch Gerontol Geriatr* 53, no. 2 (Sep–Oct 2011): e158–63. doi: 10.1016/j.archger.2010.08.004. Epub 2010 Sep 17.

29. Massachusetts General Hospital, "How to Lower Risk for Beta-Amyloid Accumulation," *Mind, Mood & Memory* 11, no. 9 (2015): 4.

Chapter 4: Every Day Is the Best Day

1. Nancy L. Mace and Peter V. Rabins, *The 36-Hour Day: A Family Guide for People Who Have Alzheimer's Disease, Related Dementias, and Memory Loss* (Baltimore: The Johns Hopkins University Press, 2011), 384.

2. Alan D Wolfelt, "Exploring Complicated Mourning: Sudden Death and Trauma Loss," seminar presented at Hospice of Davidson County, Lexington, NC, October 21, 2015.

3. Alzheimer's Society, "Dementia and the Brain," Factsheet 456LP, last reviewed September 2014, https://www.alzheimers.org.uk/site/scripts/documents_info.php?documentID=114.

4. Juebin Huang, "Brain Dysfunction by Location," Neurologic Disorders, Merck Manuals Professional Edition, http://www.merckmanuals.com/home/brain,-spinal-cord,-and-nerve-disorders/brain-dysfunction/brain-dysfunction-by-location.

5. J. Riley McCarten, "Clinical evaluation of early cognitive symptoms," *Clin Geriatr Med* 29, no. 4 (2013): 791–807. doi: 10.1016/j.cger.2013.07.005.

6. Eric H. Chudler, "Lobes of the Brain," Neuroscience for Kids, https://faculty.washington.edu/chudler/lobe.html.

7. Cedars-Sinai Medical Center, "Neurons in Brain's 'Face Recognition Center' Respond Differently in Patients with Autism," press release Nov. 20, 2013, http://cedars-sinai.edu/About-Us/News/News-Releases-2013/ Neurons-in-Brains-Face-Recognition-Center-Respond-Differently-in-Patients-With-Autism.aspx.

8. Mace and Rabins, *The 36-Hour Day*, 385.

9. Karen Leigh, "Communicating with Unconscious Patients," *Nursing Times* 97, no. 48 (2001): 35.

10. Geoffrey Lean, "'Locked in a coma, I could hear people talking around me,'" *The Telegraph*, November 24, 2009, http://www.telegraph.co.uk/news/health/6638155/Locked-in-a-coma-I-could-hear-people-talking-around-me.html.

11. Joanne Koenig Coste, *Learning to Speak Alzheimer's: A Groundbreaking Approach for Everyone Dealing with the Disease* (New York: Mariner Books, 2004), 7.

12. John Riehl, "Alzheimer's patients can still feel the emotion long after the memories have vanished," IowaNow, September 24, 2014, http://now.uiowa.edu/2014/09/alzheimers-patients-can-still-feel-emotion-long-after-memories-have-vanished.

13. Edmarie Guzma et al., "Feelings Without Memory in Alzheimer Disease," *Cogn Behav Neurol* 27 (2014): 117–129.

14. Paul R. McHugh, foreword to *The 36-Hour Day*, xviii.

15. Gary Chapman, *The 5 Love Languages®: The Secret to Love that Lasts* (Chicago: Northfield Publishing, 2015), 31, 44.

16. Sophie Behrman et al., "Considering the senses in the diagnosis and management of dementia," *Maturitas* 77, no. 4 (2014): 305–310.

17. Jolene Brackey, *Creating Moments of Joy for Persons with Alzheimer's or Dementia*, 4th Edition (West Lafayette, IN: Purdue University Press, 2007), 13.

18. Chapman, *The 5 Love Languages®*, 79.

19. Gary Chapman and Ross Campbell, *The 5 Love Languages® of Children* (Chicago: Northfield Publishing, 2012), 8.

Chapter 5: Facilitating Love

1. Nancy L. Mace and Peter V. Rabins, *The 36-Hour Day: A Family Guide for People Who Have Alzheimer's Disease, Related Dementias, and Memory Loss* (Baltimore: The Johns Hopkins University Press, 2011), 17–18.

2. Merriam-Webster Dictionary, "language," http://www.merriam-webster.com/dictionary/language.

3. Alzheimer's Foundation of America, "Music," http://www.alzfdn.org/educationandcare/musictherapy.html.

4. Jonathan Graff-Radford, "How can music help people who have Alzheimer's disease?", www.mayoclinic.org/diseases-conditions/alzheimers-disease/expert-answers/music-and-alzheimers/faq-20058173.

5. L.E. Maguire et al., "Participation in Active Singing Leads to Cognitive Improvements in Individuals with Dementia," *J Am Geriatr Soc.* 63 (2015): 815–816. doi: 10.1111/jgs.13366.

6. Alissa Sauer, "5 Reasons Why Music Boosts Brain Activity," Alzheimers.net (blog), July 21, 2014, http://www.alzheimers.net/2014-07-21/why-music-boosts-brain-activity-in-dementia-patients/.

7. Nicholas R., Simmons-Stern et al., "Music as a memory enhancer in patients with Alzheimer's disease,"*Neuropsychologia* 48, no. 10 (2010): 3164–3167. Published online May 7, 2010. doi: 10.1016/j.neuropsychologia.2010.04.033.

8. Conan Milner, "Opera Singer Turned Neuroscientist Uses Music as Medicine for Dementia, Autism, and More,"*Epoch Times*, November 26, 2015 (last updated May 25, 2016), http://www.theepochtimes.com/n3/1905111-opera-singer-turned-neuroscientist-uses-music-as-medicine-for-dementia-autism-and-more/.

9. John Schmid, "Music Therapy for Alzheimer's," Best Alzheimer's Products, November 4, 2014, http://www.best-alzheimers-products.com/music-therapy-alzheimers.html.

10. Loretta Quinn, "A Music Therapist Looks at Dementia," Best Alzheimer's Products, November 6, 2014, www.best-alzheimers-products.com/music-therapist-looks-dementia.html.

11. Earl Henslin, *This is Your Brain on Joy: How the New Science of Happiness Can Help You Feel Good and Be Happy* (Nashville: Thomas Nelson, 2008), 47–48.

12. Mary Ellen Geist, "The Healing Power of Music," *AARP Bulletin*, July/August 2015.

13. Mary Mittelman, "NYU Caregiver/Family Counseling Intervention," address at Wake Forest School of Medicine Dementia Counseling and Care Conference, Winston-Salem, NC, May 8–10, 2014.

14. Sylvia Sörensen et al., "How effective are interventions with caregivers? An updated meta-analysis," *Gerontologist* 42, no. 3 (2002): 356–372.

Chapter 6: Stories of *Hesed*

1. Gary Chapman, *The 5 Love Languages®: The Secret to Love that Lasts* (Chicago: Northfield Publishing, 2010), 40.

2. Gary Chapman, *The 5 Love Languages®*, 44.

3. Mayo Clinic, "Lewy body dementia," http://www.mayoclinic.org/diseases-conditions/lewy-body-dementia/basics/definition/con-20025038.

4. Lewy Body Dementia Association, "Capgras Syndrome in DLB Associated with Anxiety and Hallucinations," https://www.lbda.org/content/capgras-syndrome-dlb-associated-anxiety-and-hallucinations-0.

5. Alzheimer's Association, "Frontotemporal Dementia," http://www.alz.org/dementia/fronto-temporal-dementia-ftd-symptoms.asp.

6. The Association for Frontotemporal Degeneration, "FAQ," http://www .theaftd.org/life-with-ftd/newly-diagnosed/faq.

7. University of California, San Francisco, "Frontotemporal Dementia Overview," http://memory.ucsf.edu/ftd/overview.

8. Gary Chapman, *The 5 Love Languages*®, 151–158.

Chapter 7: Voices of Experience

1. Jennifer Ghent-Fuller, *Thoughtful Dementia Care: Understanding the Dementia Experience*, 1st Edition (Thoughtful Dementia Care, Inc., 2012), Kindle location page 166.

Chapter 8: The Journey No One Wants to Take

1. Alzheimer's Association, "2016 Alzheimer's Disease Facts and Figures," http:// www.alz.org/documents_custom/2016-facts-and-figures.pdf, 17, 23, 56.

Appendix A: 40 Ways to Say "I Love You" in Middle- and Late-Stage Dementia

1. Rebecca G. Logsdon and Linda Teri, "The Pleasant Events Schedule-AD: Psychometric Properties and Relationship to Depression and Cognition in Alzheimer's Disease Patients," *The Gerontologist* 37, no. 1 (1997): 40–45.

2. Adapted from *Creating Moments of Joy for Persons with Alzheimer's or Dementia*, 4th edition by Jolene Brackey. Used by permission of Purdue University Press.

Appendix B: For Those Who Want to Know More

1. Steven A. Goldman, "Brain," Merck Manual, Consumer Version, https:// www.merckmanuals.com/home/brain,-spinal-cord,-and-nerve-disorders/ biology-of-the-nervous-system/brain.

2. Brain Injury Alliance of Utah, "Cognitive Skills of the Brain," http://biau.org/ about-brain-injuries/cognitive-skills-of-the-brain/.

3. J. Riley McCarten, "Clinical evaluation of early cognitive symptoms," *Clin Geriatr Med.* 29, no. 4 (2013):791-807. doi: 10.1016/j.cger.2013.07.005.

4. Alzheimer's Association, "Posterior Cortical Atrophy," http://www.alz.org/ dementia/posterior-cortical-atrophy.asp.

5. Bonnie Badenoch, *Being a Brain-Wise Therapist: A Practical Guide to Interpersonal Neurobiology*, 1st edition (New York: W. W. Norton & Company, 2008).

6. Attachment & Emotion Regulation: Brain-Based Therapy and Practical Neuroscience, Audio CD, PESI, Inc. CMI Education. Copyright 2012.

7. Alzheimer's Association, "2016 Alzheimer's Disease Facts and Figures," http:// www.alz.org/documents_custom/2016-facts-and-figures.pdf, 7.

Acknowledgments

We were not very far along in this project before we realized that, like care partnering, writing a book is also a team sport. Many people encouraged us and helped us along the way, and we would like to thank them:

For reading all or parts of the manuscript, catching typos, sharing insights, and offering suggestions that truly improved our work:

Erin Washington
Chris Barr
Leah Shaw
Karolyn Chapman
Dwight Harris
Carrie Shaw
Chris Wynne
Samantha Rogers, PA-C

For enthusiastically supporting us with encouraging texts, emails, cards, kindnesses, and prayers:

Eileen Hamilton	Dee F. Johnson	Linda C. Hill
Sandra Swartz	Joan Long	Anne Wagner
Beth Lineberry	Dr. Elizabeth A. May	Bob Long
Beth Yancey	Joe Lineberry	Don Bell
Dwight Harris	Jeannie Yarbrough	Cynthia Baldwin
Janet Parrish	Debbie Gilreath	Andrea Buczynski
Sheri Bowman	Denise Tate	

Special thanks go to Christina Hugenschmidt, PhD, and Julie Williams, MD, for generously sharing their professional expertise with us. Thanks also to our transcriptionists, Bethany Boggs, Charla Craver Posey, and Mary Benfield.

We especially want to express our sincere gratitude to the 12 care partners who candidly shared their stories with us in one-on-one interviews and/or participated in the focus group. To ensure their anonymity, we did not use their real names, but they are each personally known by us and held in highest regard. Their personal stories gave us an in-depth look into both the dementia care partner-patient relationship and the care partnering experience. Collectively, these stories comprise a unique body of qualitative research which we have sought to faithfully represent in this volume.

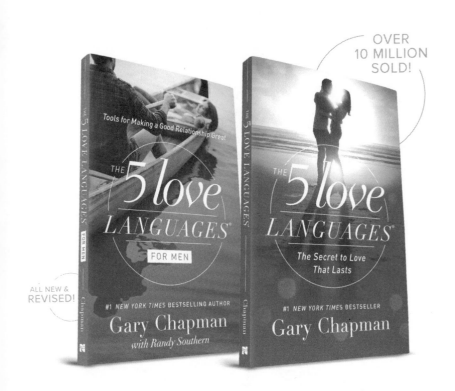

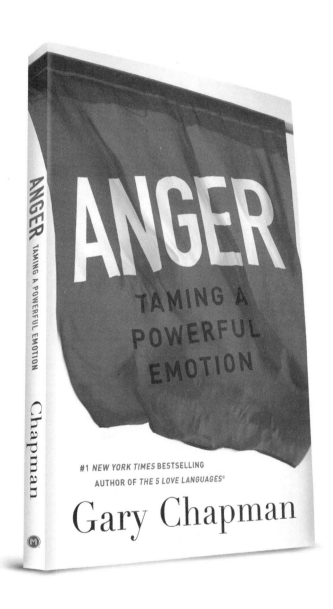

Anger is a reality of life, but it doesn't have to control our lives.
Learn how to control anger and use it for good.

WWW.5LOVELANGUAGES.COM

WHAT'S YOUR APOLOGY LANGUAGE?

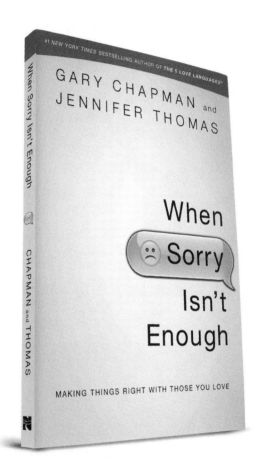

#1 *New York Times* bestselling author Gary Chapman and Jennifer Thomas have teamed up to deliver this ground-breaking study of how we give and receive apologies. It's not just a matter of will, but it's a matter of how you say, "I'm sorry" that ultimately makes things right with those you love. This book will help you discover why certain apologies clear the path for emotional healing, reconciliation, and freedom, while others fall desperately short.

WWW.5LOVELANGUAGES.COM

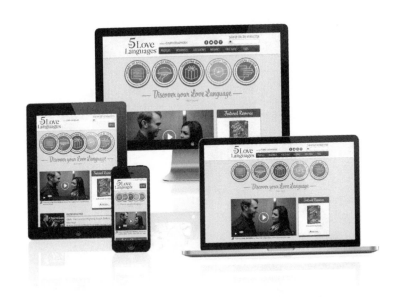
 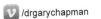